# Advance Praise for
## *Lay Down Your Guns* and Dr. Amanda Madrid

"... chronicles the life, faith, and adventures of Dr. Amanda Madrid, an indigenous Honduran missionary doctor.... riveting tales of the doctor's bold heroism in the face of adversity."
  —**Publishers Weekly**

"Dr. Amanda Madrid is a true modern-day Mother Teresa."
  —**Mark Manassee,** Senior Minister, Culver Palms Church of Christ, Los Angeles

"Dr. Amanda Madrid teaches me, gives me advice, and shows me a great model of what it means to help the poor."
  —**Gilberto Guifarro Montescleoca**, ranch owner, Catacamas, Honduras

"Dr. Amanda Madrid is a model for me and many others. Her compassion for the poor, intelligence, leadership abilities, work ethic, and ability to bridge the cultural gaps between a poor mountain community in rural Honduras and a boardroom in a large city in the USA are characteristics that set her apart."
  —**Cliff Fullerton**, M.D., M.Sc., VP, Baylor Health Care System

"Dr. Amanda Madrid is one of the most inspiring persons I know. It is one thing to talk about issues and needs in a society or country and yet another thing to actively do something by setting the example and serving the people with an inspired heart—as Dr. Madrid does. She is called by God and has walked by faith to impact many generations in her country of Honduras. A humble charismatic servant, Dr. Madrid has an amazing determination to serve God and love people through His grace. I smile every time I think of Dr. Madrid. She brings joy in a world of suffering."
  —**Mike Miller**, Fellowship of Christian Athletes, Atlanta, Georgia

"In his latest book, *Lay Down Your Guns*, Greg Taylor tells the story of Dr. Amanda Madrid's work in the mountain jungles of Honduras where warring cartels traffic not only illicit drugs but also fear and death. Well researched by Taylor through personal interviews and on site visits, the story of this brave doctor's faith, compassion and bravery in the mountains of Honduras will both inspire and humble you. This book is a must read for those of us who live in a land of safety and plenty where our faith is seldom challenged with life and death choices like Dr. Madrid makes daily.

    —**Robert D. Garland**, Paradigm Risk Management in Tulsa, Oklahoma

"Dr. Madrid lives between two worlds. She has an amazing ability to connect with people, including the most undervalued people in the community. She inspires and motivates me to be a better person. She is one of my heroes."

    —**Linda Clark**, Leadership Corp, Sarasota, Florida

"Through determination, passion, vision, and ultimately faith, Dr. Madrid has impacted the lives of countless people. Her life and work is an inspiration to me, and I believe her story will move anyone who hears it."

    —**Shane Jackson**, President, Jackson Healthcare, Alpharetta, Georgia

# LAY DOWN
# YOUR GUNS

# LAY DOWN YOUR GUNS

## One Doctor's Battle for Hope and Healing in Honduras

### Greg R. Taylor

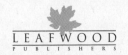

LEAFWOOD
PUBLISHERS

# LAY DOWN YOUR GUNS
*One Doctor's Battle for Hope and Healing in Honduras*

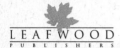

Copyright 2013 by Greg R. Taylor

ISBN 978-0-89112-342-2
LCCN 2013023024

Printed in the United States of America

Scripture references from King James Version

Spanish Scripture references from Nueva Versión Internacional.

LIBRARY OF CONGRESS CATALOGING-IN-PUBLICATION DATA
Taylor, Greg R.
  Lay down your guns : one doctor's battle for hope and healing in the honduran wild west / Greg R. Taylor.
     pages cm
  ISBN 978-0-89112-342-2
1. Madrid, Amanda--Biography. 2. Physicians--Honduras--Biography. 3. Women physi-cians--Honduras--Biography. 4. Violence--Honduras. 5. Drug dealers--Honduras. I. Title.
  R483.M316T39 2013
  610.92--dc23
  [B]
                                                                    2013023024

Original cover art by Isaac Alexander
Interior text design by Sandy Armstrong

Leafwood Publishers
1626 Campus Court
Abilene, Texas 79601
1-877-816-4455 toll free

For current information about all Leafwood titles, visit our Web site:
www.leafwoodpublishers.com

13  14  15  16  17  18  /  7  6  5  4  3  2

# Contents

# Author's Note

*Lay Down Your Guns* is a work of narrative non-fiction, a true story that reads like a novel told through Dr. Amanda Madrid's point of view.

In the Prologue and Epilogue, you will read my first person account of what I witnessed in Honduras, but the rest of the book is told in third person through Amanda Madrid's perceptions of reality—from childhood till present day. This is not an official story of the organization Dr. Madrid directs. It is biography in form of a dramatic "as told memoir" about particular episodes in the doctor's life in Honduras. Many important people, organizations, and events have been omitted in order to tell this extraordinary story.

Since the story spans nearly sixty years, I attempt to faithfully recreate scenes with dialogue crafted from memories of those who were present. Where I have reason to believe someone may be sensitive to, endangered by, or hostile to being identified in the book, I use pseudonyms.[1]

The doctor's first name, Amanda, is pronounced *ah-MAHN-dah*. Madrid is pronounced like the city in Spain.

In Honduras I conducted embedded interviews in the doctor's home, in clinics, and in the mountain jungles. Fact checking was scrupulous, but I take responsibility for inevitable mistakes. Where you may notice inaccuracies, I humbly ask your forgiveness and welcome your correspondence about things you like or dislike about the book.

---

[1] The following names in the story are pseudonyms: Bernardo, Sam, Bill, Julio, Rodrigo, Emilio, Maynor, Diego, Tamara, Veronica, Michael, Pedro, Fernando Rodriguez, Mario Hernandez, Doña Lola, Manny, any reference to family names of Mendoza and Salazar.

I did not set out to write hagiography—a biography with an angelic halo. Instead, I set out to write a true story well told about a singularly fascinating person who inspires us to live justly, humbly, and mercifully.

Greg R. Taylor
August 2013

*For Anna*

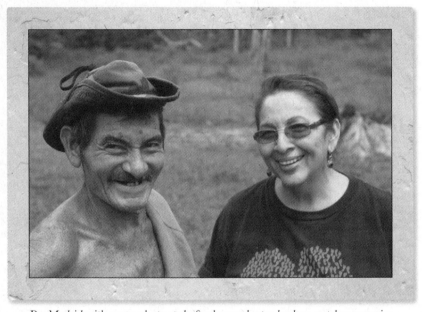

*Dr. Madrid with a man she treated after he was beaten by drug cartel mercenaries.*

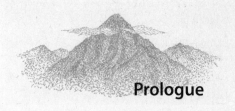

# AGUA CALIENTE, HONDURAS

*October 19, 2012*

**Dr. Amanda Madrid's driver guided us in a Landcruiser on a narrow horse path in the Cuyamel River Valley of Central Honduras, where Dr. Madrid had just spoken to** frightened medical personnel. More drug-cartel connected murders had been committed in the region, panic led to five clinics closing temporarily, and medical workers needed a plan from the doctor to care for pregnant women and sick children.

My purpose for traveling with the doctor was to see her in action as background for this book, but when two armed Honduran men stepped from behind a thick stand of eucalyptus trees into the path of our vehicle, what she did next became vital to understanding Dr. Amanda Madrid.

Both men were camo'd up, armed with Glocks and AK-47s. One man guarded the bend in the road ahead, while the other stepped directly in front of the vehicle. In Honduras, police stop cars at roadblocks everyday, but these men were neither police patrols nor military, so adrenaline surged and worst-case scenarios flashed to mind.

Driver Don Gil—a fifty-eight-year-old Honduran who bowed with his head against the steering wheel before we left, praying for our safety and success—applied the brakes and stopped the vehicle, but he kept the diesel engine percolating, ready to make necessary moves to escape, even if furiously in reverse.

"Get down in the floorboard," I told my sixteen-year-old daughter, who had come with me to Honduras as my assistant. She did not hunch down but focused on the armed men, wanting to know what was going on. I didn't know. All I could tell her was we were in a village called *Agua Caliente.* Hot Water.

To my surprise, the door of the Landcruiser opened, and Dr. Madrid reached for her calendar book and pen.

What was she doing? Why were these armed men stopping us and why was Dr. Madrid getting out? Why couldn't Don Gil simply wave, point to the Predisan logo on the vehicle—the equivalent in this region of a Red Cross symbol—and drive on?

"I know these guys," Dr. Madrid said.

Really? Dr. Madrid knows heavily armed men on remote roads in the mountains? Granted, for twenty-five years Dr. Madrid had treated nearly every person in this Cuyamel River Valley region and indeed seemed to know everyone, but armed thugs?

Dr. Madrid stuck the pen through the bun of her hair, stepped out of the vehicle onto the dirt road, and strode toward the first man in the road not cautiously but boldly. She smiled—the only time wrinkles appeared on her face; you would expect more visible wear from a fifty-six-year-old female doctor, traveled as she is—and held out her right hand toward the man.

With her left hand Dr. Madrid brushed back a wisp of auburn hair, pushed up her glasses that had slipped down because of sweat, and her long earrings gently rocked beneath her strong jaws as she came to a stop in front of the man about twenty feet in front of us.

The armed man stuffed his Glock in the backside waistband of his pants, then shook hands with the doctor.

Dr. Madrid was the only one of the five in the vehicle courageous enough to go toe to toe with these men, they in their combat boots, and she in her blazing red high heels. Honduran men seem to respect the doctor because she doesn't speak like most Honduran women, in deference to men, but looks with her brown eyes directly into theirs. She doesn't dress like a typical Honduran woman in a skirt, but she wears jeans and high heels.

Dr. Madrid is no ordinary Honduran woman. The people who work with her say, *"Tiene los pantalones bien puestos.* She wears the pants well." There's slang in Spanish that they also say about her, and it means figuratively that "she is a tough leader," but the literal words wouldn't pass for good taste in genteel company. They say about her *"Tiene huevos.* She has eggs." And in Latin America, they're *not* referring to the female kind of eggs.

Over the past few years, Dr. Madrid has had to wear the pants because this wasn't the first time she'd gone toe to toe with armed men pointing their Kalashnikovs at her—men, who with their small-scale war of land grabbing, revenge, jealousy, and drugs, were swiftly destabilizing the medical clinics that had for twenty-five years served the people of Olancho, a state known as the "Wild West of Honduras." The violence between two warring gangs destabilized the clinics and threatened the health of residents in the mountain jungles. After decades of having no access to health care, mountain residents enjoyed a network of small clinics for prenatal care, safe delivery of babies, and treatment of infectious diseases, but now all that was in jeopardy.

Dr. Madrid told the man on the road the problem she had explained to me: "People are afraid to transport the sick at night because cars are being stopped; thugs are beating people, stealing from them, threatening them. A pregnant woman died in childbirth recently because her family waited till the next morning to transport her to the hospital. A young girl bitten by a snake also died because her family was afraid to go anywhere at night in this region," Dr. Madrid said.

"My staff is developing an evacuation plan in the five mountain clinics to take sick children, adults, and pregnant women out to hospitals in case of emergencies," Dr. Madrid told the man. I could see veins bulging in the doctor's neck as she spoke. I learned the man's name but will use a pseudonym, Diego Salazar.

Diego listened then told the doctor he's defending his village against a drug cartel buying up land and cattle to launder money and to clear a path for transporting drugs through this region.

She did not argue with his point but made clear she doesn't want Diego or anyone stopping Predisan vehicles when medical workers transport the sick for care. Dr. Madrid gestured with her finger nearly touching his chest. Diego wore a dark button-down shirt, camouflage cargo pants, combat boots, and next to the Glock, clipped to his belt, he had a high-powered two-way radio.

Twenty-five years ago, Dr. Madrid rode a horse into these mountains to heal the sick, pray for them, show them the love of Jesus she had come to know and serve. When she rode in with a team of Hondurans and North Americans, they dreamed of establishing medical clinics in the rugged mountain jungles of Olancho, and over time that dream would come true through an organization named Predisan, a word meant to describe the group's activities, an invented Spanish two-word splice meaning "to preach and to heal."

Dr. Madrid started coming to these mountains when thirty-year-old Diego was a young boy. She saw Diego playing soccer on a little field with cut tree limbs lashed together for goals, and she thought he was a fast and skilled player. When she met Diego and his brothers in the clinics, taught them in the Bible study meetings she also conducted, she saw a friendly, handsome boy who seemed to like guns and often strapped one on his back when he went with his uncle to prospect for gold.

She knew Diego's family to be good and regular folks who were not killers, not thugs who got mixed up with narco gangs or even battled against them. Never did the doctor imagine, however, that this little boy named Diego whom she treated in clinics would grow up to be like this: defending his life and village from a drug cartel that has made this region its newest bridge for drug traffic from South to North America. Diego had spent time in the army and looked the part, but fighting the cartel mercenaries wore on him, so he drank and took drugs to take the edge off the stress.

At one point, a gang of thugs occupied the command center of the clinic network, and Dr. Madrid refused to allow this trespassing and desecration of the mission. She accompanied the police on a raid, and the thugs fled from the clinic headquarters. With the violent men still at large in the region, however, fear gripped the staff members of the clinics, because their own family members were involved, endangered. Some refused to work, and those from cities returned, where—ironically—they felt more safe. The health and well-being of people depended on these rural mountain clinics, but now fear bled into worsening health for pregnant women giving birth to more sickly babies with fathers who were more preoccupied with their feud than raising crops, or children for that matter.

Out the side window of the Landcruiser, I saw Diego's family ranch. Coconut palms grew next to the house, leaning over and shading it. A mountain peak not far behind the house towered like a giant backdrop in a beautiful painting. A horse tromped along a slack wire fence lining the overgrown path. On the property a pond stagnated where a once thriving fish farm was overgrown with weeds, the fish belly up and decaying in rancid water. A grenade blast left a car-sized hole in the roof and shattered red roofing tiles covered the grass in front of the house. The front porch support poles looked like a beaver had chewed them. When they ran out of ammo, the attackers tried to hack down the poles to make the house fall, and they did so with a dull axe. Many of the family members who once lived here peacefully were dead or had left the village, or remained on the run, like Diego. Diego's wife and children had long ago left for the north coast of Honduras.

"I'm innocent. They killed my brother," Diego told Dr. Madrid. As Diego spoke, Dr. Madrid leaned in to listen, pulling the pen from her hair to take notes in her journal.

"They're hunting me for protecting Agua Caliente from these bad guys who are trying to take our land. I did not do anything."

He repeated again and again his innocence.

"I want to get some evidence for the police so they will know who did this to your houses," Dr. Madrid said.

She asked about the radio he was holding, and Diego told the doctor that the two-way radio was his now, that he'd found it after the mercenaries had come to destroy the homes of Diego's family. They'd dropped the radio when they torched and blew up the houses.

Dr. Madrid thought if she got the radio from Diego, prosecutors could use it for evidence in court. She'd seen it work with other murder cases. One thug who had murdered many people in the mountain jungles went to jail because families of the victims amassed evidence against him and submitted it to the police and courts. Dr. Madrid urged Diego to do the same, to give up evidence so they could convict these guys.

But Diego was reluctant. With the radio he could hear his enemy's movements, whether or not they are coming for him. The radio transmits for miles on a low-wave frequency. He admitted, however, that the battery was now depleted and he did not have a charger. Why not give up the radio now for evidence? He gripped the radio, rolled it in his hands, placed it back in the waistband of his trousers.

"I've been shot ten times," Diego said, and he took off his shirt to reveal scars covering his back. He lifted his pant leg to show scars on this leg. One bullet was still lodged under his skin. The scars were fresh but healed over. Diego had a moustache and days of beard growth on his neck and chin only, and his cheeks and sideburns looked shaved clean. Though he'd been in hiding in other houses or in the forest, it was obvious that someone had been feeding him. He wasn't fat but thick and strong, of medium height and brown wavy hair pushed back in a style you would expect if he were a stage singer named Diego.

Dr. Madrid examined the scars and a bullet still lodged in his arm. Then she turned toward the Landcruiser and motioned for me to come with my camera. I fumbled to put on the correct lens, got out and walked to them.

Diego held out his hand and I held out mine, and we shook and greeted one another in Spanish. When he learned I am from the United States, he said he had lived in New Jersey eight years, working on a tree service crew, going out on limbs. He didn't say what I expected someone to say in that situation, that he liked my country and would return to visit friends someday. He was not going back to the United States. He said whatever happens he would stay in the mountain jungles of Honduras to fight for his land and village.

The doctor looked at me and pointed to my camera. "Why don't you take some pictures of his wounds?"

I aimed the camera at Diego, he muttered something I didn't understand, then Dr. Madrid turned to me and said, "Don't get his face in the photo."

I clicked off two dozen photos. Then he held his arm up by his face to reveal what looked like a marble under his skin, as if to invite me to photograph his face, regardless of what he'd said. I took a photo of his arm, and because I was rattled, uncertain if I'd see Diego again, and wanted to tell you what he looks like, I clicked the shutter to capture his face.

To keep Diego's wish and protect his life, I would not publish the photograph. I looked at the photo on the back of my camera and smiled back at him. The photo showed Diego with something between a smile and a smirk, holding up his arm with the bullet lodged under his skin. The lines around his soft brown eyes are either smiling or yawning crevices from lack of sleep, I couldn't tell which.

"Those guys coming after me are buying up land for safe passage for their goods, and they're buying cattle—they have big houses," Diego said.

"The police can't arrest you for having a big house; you need to give up the radio as evidence and talk to the police yourself to give them information that could lead to their arrest," Dr. Madrid told Diego.

Diego persisted in his claim of innocence, said he's living like a fox on the run and burrowing in at night like an armadillo.

"I've been up the Patuca River, and I know that area you are talking about, where they run drugs and land planes on airstrips they've built there. Even if I go up there with the police they need evidence to make arrests," Dr. Madrid said.

Diego laughed. "You're thinking of going up there! You'll never get out of there alive!"

"No, no, I'm not planning to go up there now," Dr. Madrid said, and she laughed, a hearty, nasally cackle. Diego breathed a sigh and laughed again.

"Diego, you've been shot many times and you are still alive, so God may have a purpose for you in this community—for peace not war! But how can God use you for peace if you don't submit to him? We taught you the word of God when you were a child, when you and your brother, Emilio, came to our church," Dr. Madrid said.

Diego listened to what the doctor said, but I wondered if he truly believed that peace was an option. He seemed bent not only on defending his village but also on avenging the blood of his murdered brother.

Dr. Madrid ended their conversation exactly the way she did every time she pleaded with armed men like Diego. She looked at Diego with glistening brown eyes and said, "Lay down your guns."

I went back to the Landcruiser, but the doctor and Diego talked a few more minutes. As I turned and watched what she did next, I found the extraordinary scene hard to fathom. So, from a distance, I took what turned out to be a blurry photo of Dr. Madrid and Diego standing in the road. In the photo, Diego's head is bowed and Dr. Madrid has her hand on Diego's shoulder—she is praying with him.

I'd witnessed uncommon bravery and spirituality in one person, but I was also perplexed. I wanted to know: Who is Dr. Amanda Madrid? And how did she, against all odds, become such a creative, spiritual, and courageous doctor?

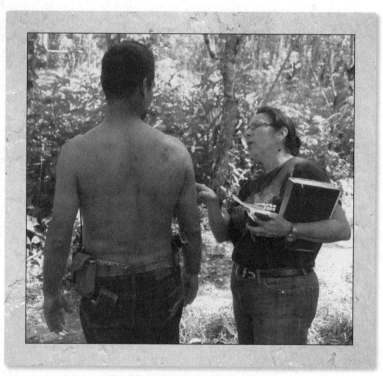

*Dr. Madrid with Diego on the road.*

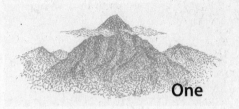

# One

# NO GUARANTEE IT CAN BE STOPPED

**Diego and his brothers—like all residents of the Cuyamel River Valley—came to expect that Dr. Madrid would not leave until she had prayed for them.**

For the moment Diego's shoulders dropped slightly; he stopped taking second-by-second inventory of his surroundings and bowed his head to receive Dr. Madrid's prayer.

"Lord, I know you love Diego and all of his family. He's not a bad person. He needs to put down his guns, to forgive. All these bullet wounds! All these scars! Like the scars on your body, dear Jesus! Diego must be alive for a purpose. Help him find that purpose, Holy Father," the doctor prayed.

After she ended the prayer, Dr. Madrid embraced Diego long, as if she were his mother, and they said goodbye. Diego moved to the side of the road so the vehicle could pass, and he rejoined his friend who had been standing guard with his AK-47.

Diego waved as the Landcruiser passed close by him on the narrow trail.

The Landcruiser slipped through the thick stand of eucalyptus and pine trees on the erstwhile horse-only trail where now a few vehicles pass daily. Back on the main dirt road, the vehicle forded a stream, descending then ascending a big muddy "V" shape, then passed a boy talking on his cell phone while riding a horse up a steep rise in the dirt road.

"I'm not judging these men," Dr. Madrid said, as we descended winding mountain roads in the vehicle. "I simply want them to know that God loves them, that I love them, that Predisan cares about them. In spite of anything they are doing, I want them to know that if they have any injuries, we'll help them. I don't think judging them is my job, even though I don't approve of what they are doing, and they know that. But I feel the responsibility to talk to them about God."

Don Gil managed the winding mountain road and turned southwest on the paved highway, passing a pickup with a dozen Honduran men and women police officers riding in the bed of the truck. Don Gil slowed the vehicle near a high school where throngs of uniformed students cross the road to an eatery on the other side. In a one hour car ride back from the mountains to Catacamas, Dr. Madrid made or received a dozen phone calls on two phones—sometimes both at once—as she prepared for more meetings. She'd already missed a board conference call because of the long stop with Diego. She would ask the board chairperson's forgiveness for missing the call, for being "held up," as it were, by armed men.

Between calls Dr. Madrid recounted her dialogue with Diego.

"Diego said over and over that he is innocent, that he's just protecting his village from the narcos who want to buy land and cattle and run their drugs through there," she said.

She didn't want him to end up like so many others in the past two years. Since 2011, forty-two men and women had been killed in the mountain jungles surrounding the five Predisan clinics where the population of the region is 14,228. With a population of a small town, the murder rate for the past two years is that of a large metropolitan city.

Machetes are part of the rural Honduran culture. Rural men have long carried machetes as urbane men carry a pen and pocketknife. A farmer who does not read or write may never need a pen, but he will still need to communicate beyond words at times, and for that he has his machete. Add to these wood and steel appendages of enmity the new business of running drugs and doled out rifles and pistols and the infusion into the mountain jungles of more cash than most *campesinos* (farmers) ever held in their hands and the result is quite literally jungle law. Add resistance to the whole business by one clan of locals next to the compliance and complicity of another clan and you begin to understand something of what's happening in the mountains of Central America, in places like the Cuyamel River Valley where Dr. Madrid's team has struggled to establish a network of clinics where there was once only traditional jungle medicine.

Over the years, Dr. Madrid has spoken with traditional healers and challenged the efficacy and ethics of "drugs" they distribute, but the new worst obstacle to health in the mountain jungles is illegal drug trafficking. Drugs are often flown into airstrips that serve as drop points between the mountain clinics and the Mosquito Coast. If you are a trafficker, you can't successfully fly long distances in international airspace or over patrolled coastal waters. You must refuel. You need stopovers. You need manpower to transport "packages" by boat, horseback, or on foot to the next airstrip or open waterway. So the cartels pay a farmer ten times what he normally makes from selling a break-your-back sack of beans or corn to transport those packages. Carriers and mercenary armed guards passing through rely on local women to cook for them. The men are willing to pay the women gourmet prices for beans, corn tortillas, and a freshly killed hen. Many of the men expect more than food for the price they pay.

A farmer or trained health care worker makes only a fraction of what a "mule" can make in one trip with drugs over the mountains. Some international aid organizations working in the mountains find it increasingly difficult to train agricultural workers when a farmer makes 50,000 lempiras a year raising and selling crops, but the same farmer sees his neighbor making 500,000 lempiras as a "mule" carrying drugs.

Two other non-governmental organizations recently pulled out of their work in the mountain jungles, citing security concerns; but they were also experiencing difficulty getting people interested in their training and vocations compared to the newest vocation of packing drugs by horseback and human backs via rivers and paths through the mountains.

Dr. Madrid had no intention of pulling Predisan clinics out of the mountain jungles because of these disparities of pay, nor because dangerous men were attempting to buy loyalty, land, and anything else they wanted. Villagers relied on the clinics to survive.

About the problem of the drug trade, a Honduran university rector named Dr. Julieta Castellanos said in an October 13, 2012 *New York Times* article, "There's infiltration everywhere." And she gravely concludes in the article, "There is no guarantee it can be stopped."

The son of Dr. Castellanos was allegedly killed by police with ties to drug cartels. Dr. Madrid feels Dr. Castellanos' despondency and loss of hope about the intractable problem of the drug trade in Honduras. She also understands why poor people often turn to drug transporting and selling.

"Everyone has their price," Dr. Madrid said. "Imagine you are a police officer or health care worker, and someone offers you easy money. You are under pressure to feed your family. If you don't have ethics, don't have God in your life, you give in."

Don Gil drove the Predisan vehicle into Catacamas, returning Dr. Madrid from a half day in the mountains, from her meeting with one hundred Predisan staffers and volunteers and confrontation with Diego on the road, back to her hometown and Predisan headquarters. For the last twenty-five years, the doctor has treated someone in nearly every family in this town.

With 44,000 residents, Catacamas was surrounded by lush, green, low-slung mountains and gridded with roads ranging from paved to cobblestone to cratered gravel. The afternoon temperature was making its regular climb to the nineties and lunchtime street vendors sold *baleadas* (Honduran burritos), roasted chicken, tamales, and bananas. A few hundred meters from the police department, across the street from a soccer field, a green metal sign reading "Predisan" was bent into an "L" shape from a vehicle hitting it, and no one had bothered to bend it back in place. A rusty old phone booth next to the Predisan sign was out of commission, and teenage girls in jeans—which they would not be welcomed to wear in public a few years ago—passed in front of the defunct phone booth, talking on their cell phones while walking on the dusty shoulder of the road. Trucks lumbered by and small cars slowed down to avoid scraping bottom on the massive speed bumps.

Across from the soccer field, down the street from the police station, next to the bent green sign and the old phone booth, a small parking lot and an archway led into Predisan's *Complejo de Salud Familiar* (Family Health Clinic). The clinic was established in 1986 as the *Clinica Buen Samaritano* (Good Samaritan Clinic) in one room of a church where Dr. Madrid examined patients and where the exam room doubled as a lab—a microscope on the corner of the doctor's desk.

Today Predisan not only employs eighty staff members but also hosts up to four hundred volunteers annually who come mainly from North America to serve in the clinics. Dr. Madrid with her staff of doctors and nurses treat hundreds of patients weekly in this clinic with hacienda-style covered walkways, a central open-air garden, a chapel where the staff meets daily to pray together and ask God to help them once again preach hope to the hopeless and heal the sick. They pray, read scriptures in Spanish, and prepare themselves for the onslaught of patients.

Dr. Madrid got out of the Landcruiser still talking on the phone, and her assistant met her in the parking lot. They walked together through the archway, past the wheelchairs in the outdoor waiting area, down an outdoor covered walkway, and into a tiny office for Dr. Madrid, who supervises this and six rural health clinics, as well as an in-patient addiction treatment center called *El Centro de Rehabilitación del Paciente Adicto* (The Center for Rehabilitation of Patients with Addictions or CEREPA).

Martha, a short, smiling woman who'd worked twenty years in the clinic, stopped to say hello to the doctor. Martha was balancing a teetering stack of scrubs she had laundered.

"How is the baby?" Dr. Madrid asked Martha. "She's a little sick but growing well," Martha said of her ninth grandchild. "Thank you for your good work, Martha." Martha's smile widened, and she continued down the breezeway to deliver the scrubs to surgery, tenderly calling back, *"Muchas gracias."*

Every Predisan staffer—from the surgeon to the one who launders the scrubs—is expected to join the mission of Predisan: to preach and to heal. Their model is the story Jesus told of the Good Samaritan, and they continue to use the clinic name, *Clinica Buen Samaritano*. The evangelist and physician, St. Luke, recounts the story Jesus told: A man was beaten by robbers and left for dead on the road. Religious leaders cut the victim a wide berth because to touch him would make them ritually unclean and temporarily ineligible for priestly duties—and their livelihood. Then a man from Samaria, a place those religious leaders thought was full of sinners and outcasts, saw the man, took pity on him, bound up his wounds, put him on his own donkey, took him to an inn, and paid for the victim's treatment.

Luke says that after Jesus tells this story he asks an expert in the law which one of the men traveling on the road was a good neighbor to the man. The expert replied, "The one who had mercy on him." Then Jesus said, "Go and do likewise," which is what the staff of *Clinica Buen Samaritano* have agreed to do.

Dr. Madrid walked down the hall to check an x-ray of a patient. In the radiology department she asked the tech, Hector, if the x-ray was ready. A local power outage shut down the x-ray machine, delaying the process, but the film was nearly developed.

She used the delay to chat with Hector. Dr. Madrid and Hector met in 1988 when *Clinica Buen Samaritano* had just begun, and he was trained as one of the first volunteer health care workers. Dr. Madrid recruited Hector as a volunteer for his home area, El Coyote.

Like Martha, who was in charge of the medical clinic laundry, Hector had given most of his career to the mission of Predisan.

The hum of the x-ray machine and sterile environment of the clinic contrasted with the austere small clinic where Hector worked in El Coyote. That clinic was an adobe brick building with a few rooms to dispense free medical care to his long-time neighbors. Dr. Madrid had taught hundreds of men and women like Hector who then received further training to become advanced health care employees.

The trained staff has responded to human suffering in the Honduran mountain jungles: pregnant women needing pre- and post-natal care, children who need immunizations, and people with injuries from fights or job-related accidents. From the earnest staff, the steady stream of patients finding relief and care, and the orderly environment of the clinic, it's clear that Predisan takes seriously the mandate of Jesus to preach and to heal. They act on the belief that God has a preferential concern for the poor. Because many cannot or will not travel to the central clinic, Dr. Madrid helped establish outposts in the mountains.

The *Clinica Buen Samaritano* and the rural clinics cooperate to provide a range of medical, psychological, and spiritual care for patients, like Valerie, a teenager in Catacamas.

One day Valerie and her friend Tamara were walking home from school in Catacamas when boys in a car stopped to offer them a ride. Each girl thought the other girl knew someone in the car. The boys were handsome with a cool car, so the girls agreed, got in, and told the boys where they lived. Minutes later, the car sped past Valerie's house, where they'd asked to be dropped off.

"Do you know any of these guys?" Valerie whispered to Tamara.

"No, do you?" Tamara replied.

"No."

Valerie and Tamara inhaled but didn't seem to exhale. The car stopped in front of a cantina and the young men ushered the girls inside, where they bought them sodas with alcohol or a drug added.

Hours later, Valerie and Tamara woke up in a strange place; next to their handbags was a total of 5,000 lempiras, and the boys were gone. They had raped both girls. But what was the money? Did the boys feel remorse? Was this hush money? The money was ten times what men paid prostitutes. Were they drug dealers? The girls heads were spinning with confusion.

Valerie and Tamara went outside to get their bearings and walked to their homes. Valerie lived in Catacamas with her older sister. Her mother lived in the United States. Though traumatized, Valerie told no one what happened, until many weeks later when she thought she was pregnant. She immediately told Tamara. Then Valerie told her older sister about the guys in the car, the drinks, the rape, the 5,000 lempiras, and the possible pregnancy, but Valerie's sister didn't believe her story.

"Go and get the boy who got you pregnant," Valerie's sister told her.

Valerie wanted to kill herself. Not only did her sister not believe the story, she also wanted her out of the house.

So Valerie called a friend, Michael, a boy who had a crush on her in their high school. Maybe he would help her find a way to kill herself, help her find a gun, a knife, pills, anything. She didn't want to live, didn't know how she would take care of a baby. All her hopes of getting a high school diploma were gone. And wouldn't her mother kill her anyway when she saw her in this condition? What was the purpose of living now? She was distraught when she reached her friend's house.

Valerie and Michael talked for a long time about what had happened, about her problems, and the teenage boy had compassion on her. "If you want I can take you to my grandparents' village," Michael said.

A few days later Valerie and Michael went to the village of his grandparents. The two teens were accustomed to city life, so village life seemed harder. Valerie cooked over an open fire, and Michael helped tend to crops and animals. After a few weeks, however, Valerie and Michael decided to stay through the end of the pregnancy.

As they passed the days in the village, Michael told Valerie he would help her take care of the baby. Valerie didn't know if she wanted that, and she was afraid of having a baby who looked like one of the boys who raped her. But the baby wouldn't look like Michael, who by this time had convinced his family—mostly by saying little and allowing them to assume—that the pregnancy was his doing. They both planned not to return to school but to build a house in the mountains and stay.

Valerie went to one of the Predisan clinics in the mountains. When Valerie hinted at the possibility of abortion, the health care worker told her she ought to talk with Dr. Amanda Madrid. She agreed.

An appointment was set and Dr. Madrid went to the village where Michael and Valerie were staying. Dr. Madrid's first task was to address questions that patients like Valerie might have, though they may not voice them all: Does rape justify having an abortion? Would an abortion further add to her feelings of shame and defilement? Is abortion a sin? Dr. Madrid pointed Valerie away from the brutal option of abortion, even though a pregnancy as a result of rape is one of the most emotionally difficult kinds of pregnancies to carry to term.

"How is Michael treating you?" Dr. Madrid asked.

"Very well," Valerie said. "He's very kind." Michael did not try to take advantage of Valerie in her vulnerability; he stayed his distance and respected her.

She talked to Valerie about the difficulties of raising a child, being a mother, how a baby develops to term, and how she would need to stay healthy.

Appointments with Dr. Madrid were more than pre-natal care for Valerie and her baby, but they were also healing visits for her soul after rape and distance from her family.

Another appointment was made for Valerie to come into the Good Samaritan Clinic for an ultrasound. X-ray techs could have done the ultrasound, but Dr. Madrid wanted to do this one personally for this scared teenager. Her sister had kicked her out, her mother remained in the United States, and Michael's mother had not warmed up to her. Dr. Madrid was not only a doctor but also a strong mother figure who gave Valerie confidence that she would make it through this.

Valerie delivered her baby in one of the Predisan clinics, and Michael began caring for the child as if he were the biological father.

Raising a baby together was hard for Michael and Valerie, and not all family members supported them. Michael's mother and grandmother suspected something was different about their relationship, and as the baby boy grew older, Michael's mother grew distant from Valerie. The tension spread to Michael and Valerie and they began to argue often and became very unhappy. A mountain clinic nurse told a Predisan chaplain that a family in her village could benefit from counseling with him.

The chaplain made an appointment to meet with Michael, Valerie, and their six-month-old baby.

"How have you been doing with the baby?"

"Good," Valerie said, and Michael agreed.

"What is the biggest problem you face in your home?"

"I want to be close to Valerie and the baby but there's a problem," Michael said.

"What sort of problem?"

Michael hesitated. He didn't want to tell their secret to the chaplain and embarrass Valerie. He shook his head side to side and waved it off. It was nothing. They didn't need to talk about it.

The chaplain waited and in the awkward silence looked at Michael.

"Well, uh, it's my mother," Michael finally said.

"What about her?"

"She is—she's distanced herself from Valerie and it seems like she doesn't approve of her or us as a couple."

The chaplain sent a messenger for Michael's mother, asking her to come to the clinic to talk. When she arrived, the chaplain talked with her about her multiple roles as mother, mother-in-law, and grandmother. He said love connects them all and that Michael, Valerie, and the baby all needed her support. When asked what she felt, Michael's mother said that she liked Valerie, but she wanted the couple to financially support themselves. The couple had tried to earn their keep, but they needed to do more to bring in money. So they decided Michael and Valerie would start a small restaurant in their village to support themselves. Though the money they made was not much, the effort itself improved family relationships.

Counseling and pre-natal care are two examples of the holistic elements of care Predisan provides, but sometimes Dr. Madrid's work is simply to do what's needed in the moment.

One day when Dr. Madrid made rounds in the mountain clinics to check on patients, some men asked the doctor to come see their friend who had been shot in the leg. When she arrived at the house where the injured man was, Dr. Madrid examined him. The bullet was lodged in his thigh but was visible. She told the man and his friends he should go to the hospital.

The men said to Dr. Madrid, "No hospital! Do what you can."

"How did this happen?" Dr. Madrid asked.

They said nothing but their facial expressions implied, *Don't ask*. Dr. Madrid normally would press for history, backstory: *Who shot you? What's going on here? What problems are you facing?* But her instincts told her these men would not reveal anything.

Dr. Madrid opened her doctor's bag to retrieve her minor surgery kit from a sterile container. She numbed the area with anesthetic, held the wound open with pins, gripped the bullet with clamps, and dislodged it. After removing the bullet, the doctor closed with sutures and bandaged the patient's leg. Having completed her task, she did not look the man's friends directly in the eyes. She packed up her sterile kit, replaced everything in the bag, and walked out.

Dr. Madrid grew tired of treating men who had injured one another in fights. She had treated many men with machete wounds. Now with more and more guns, she wondered what would happen in the mountain jungles. Sometimes she would stay as detached as extracting a bullet and walking away, but other days a girl like Valerie would walk into the clinic, and Dr. Madrid would become more than a physician but also a mother and friend.

Weeks passed following Dr. Madrid's conversation with Diego on the road in the Cuyamel River Valley, and she asked Frank Lopez, director of the five mountain clinics, "Have you seen Diego?"

Because Diego was hiding, Frank did not see him but heard reports that he was still in the region.

Then one day Frank came to the doctor with news from the mountains.

Diego had been on the run for months, dodging the drug lords, but they'd finally caught up to him.

"*Mataron a Diego.* They killed Diego."

Diego had the radio and several guns belonging to the drug traffickers. They killed Diego along with two of his friends then retrieved their radio and guns.

Dr. Madrid was distraught. She had known Diego since he was a boy. Why did his life have to turn out like this? The people she'd dedicated her life to when she rode a horse up the mountain trail many years before were dying because of turf wars, greed, and revenge.

The doctor returned to her home in Catacamas, climbed the tiled stairs, entered her second story bedroom, closed the door behind her and the curtains across the window, and fell on her bed. The news of Diego's death sent her into deep reflection and sadness. A once joyous and peaceful village now heaved with violence and dread. The doctor stayed home, sleeping, mourning, and praying for three days. What did God want from her? How could all this work in the mountains be for nothing? Would the clinics survive? Would she?

The next week, the doctor told her assistant to gather the Predisan supervisors for a meeting. Normally full of ideas for what to do next, Dr. Madrid had nothing.

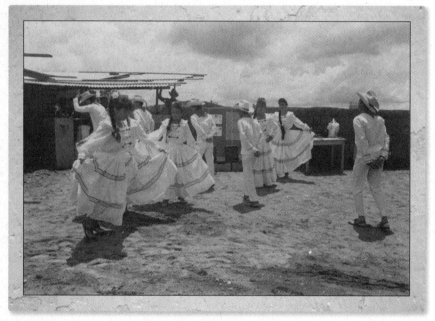

*Hondurans celebrating at a fiesta.*

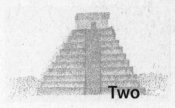

# Two

# RIDING ON THE BACK OF JESUS

**Seven-year-old Amanda was not allowed to attend the** *Viernes Santo y la Procesión y Fiesta* **(Good Friday Procession and Fiesta) that day in 1964. Amanda's father, Florencio,** Sr., forbade her from going. None of her family was to attend the festivities of Easter week in her small town near the northwestern border of Honduras. But Amanda went to the procession and fiesta anyway. José, her teenage brother, took Amanda to the *procesión* on the plaza.

"If I take you to the *procesión*, can you keep it a secret?" José asked.

Amanda knew that she needed to keep the secret from her father but how could she not tell her little brother, Florencio, Jr., all that she would see?

"Si," she said almost inaudibly, knowing even her agreement must be kept quiet, and she nodded her head and raised her eyebrows. Amanda couldn't believe her older brother, who had been studying in El Salvador, would come home for this holiday and take Amanda to the *procesión*. She had thought when she was older and could make her own decisions she would go.

The reason Florencio, Sr. forbade the family to celebrate the Catholic *procesión* was an adult concern that children had difficulty comprehending, and most adults had difficulty fathoming as well. Her father, Florencio, Sr., had not been religious for many years, but when he started attending *Templo Siloe Asamblea de Dios* (Siloam Temple Assembly of God), he heard teaching against Catholic traditions. So Florencio, Sr. declared that the Madrid family would not participate in Catholic rituals in La Jigua, the small town in the state of Copán where Amanda was born. Furthermore, none of Amanda's sisters would have a *quinceañera*, and Amanda would never be a candidate for "Queen of the Barrio." But on this Good Friday, she felt like a princess as she walked hand in hand with her brother José down the guava tree lined path from their house, past the jail house and post office and into the plaza. Townspeople had assembled to watch the procession in front of the La Jigua Cathedral, a sturdy white Spanish mission church with two bell towers framing the center arched entrance. In the middle of the wall, above the entryway, a clock displayed the official La Jigua time, pointing every midnight and noon directly to the cross above it.

Artists had decorated the main street where the *procesión* of priests and parishioners walked with statues of *Madre María y Jesucristo* (Mother Mary and Jesus Christ). On the cobblestones citizens placed colored sawdust and flowers in designs depicting the Stations of the Cross, and this carpet they believed eased the walk of Christ to the cross.

Amanda wondered why her family and church forbade such joyous colors and celebrations. Her church, *Templo Siloe Asamblea de Dios,* had no icons, no statues, nothing interesting to look at like Jesus on the shoulders of the townsmen walking the *via dolorosa* (way of grief) through the plaza. They'd draped a tunic on the shoulders of the image of Jesus; on his head they'd placed a crown of thorns. Behind those holding Jesus, another group carried an icon of Mary, adorned with flowers.

Amanda's eyes locked on the image of Mary. In her small adobe church outside the plaza, up the hill close to her home, they didn't talk much about *Madre María*, but secretly, Amanda wanted to be like Mary.

When the procession was done, townspeople went back to their selling and buying—just food on this day, no other goods would be sold—and José and Amanda went to a vendor selling sweet bread. José bought Amanda a piece of the fluffy bread covered with a red sugary coating. She let the bread melt in her mouth, but she did not eat it all. She saved some sweet bread for her toddler sister, Toñita.

José walked Amanda home where she found her next youngest sibling, Florencio, Jr., and they soon left to go out of earshot from home to talk and play. Virtually everyone in town was at the procession and fiesta but not the Madrid family and some members of their small Evangelical church. On Good Friday the family worked in the morning then went up the hill to grandma Tula's house to drink coffee and lie in the hammocks in the breezeway.

No one worked on Easter weekend. This was a Honduran version of the North American idea of "blue laws" that kept people from doing too much work on holy days when church leaders wanted congregants praying and giving their offerings to the church, and so stores closed on Good Friday.

Conventional community wisdom evolved out of this prohibition of selling. If you sold goods on crucifixion day, La Jigua residents said, at best you were selling out Jesus and at worst you were crucifying Jesus all over again. If you rode a horse on Good Friday, you were riding on the back of Jesus.

Even though her family didn't participate, Amanda's mother, Maria Antonia, had been raised Catholic, and she believed you shouldn't sell your wares or ride a horse on Good Friday. Early in their marriage, Maria Antonia urged Florencio not to ride his horse on Good Friday like a heathen, but he refused to go along with such myths. Maria Antonia prayed God would forgive Florencio for riding on the back of Jesus.

But it was the idea that you could not swim on Good Friday that most perplexed Amanda.

The weather that Good Friday in 1964 was clear and sunny, and Amanda felt like swimming, but she was forbidden to go down to the river and jump in. If she did, though, none of the regulars at the river washing clothes would see her. They were all at the fiesta.

Amanda pulled five-year-old Florencio, Jr. by the arm to a place in the trees outside their house where she could talk and no one would hear her.

"Let's go to the river to—" Amanda said to her brother, Florencio, Jr.

Florencio, Jr. heard nothing else after "river." He began running before Amanda could finish her sentence. Amanda followed him down the path.

The path to the Juile River from the Madrid house was narrow and worn, lined with bougainvillea bushes in brilliant reds and oranges and shaded by palms. As they walked, Florencio, Jr. craned his neck looking for bird's nests in the trees. Amanda and Florencio, Jr. had a running contest: the first to find a bird's nest "owned" the nest.

Butterflies fluttered above their heads like a flock of angels, floating on upward bursts of air created by the children's breezy running. The air smelled of grass and the pungent sweet smell of cows and horses grazing nearby.

They reached the bank of the Juile River and jumped on a large flat rock that felt warm and smooth to their bare feet.

"Let's put our toes in the water," Amanda said.

"No, Amanda! We can't get into the water. That's dangerous!"

Adults in La Jigua often told children, "If you swim on Good Friday, you will become a fish." Frightened by the prospect of such a metamorphosis, Florencio did not want even to touch the water on Good Friday.

"Let's just dip our toes. If that part of us becomes a fin, we'll cover it with our shoes," Amanda assured Florencio.

Amanda knew in the end Florencio would do whatever she told him to do—it was simply a matter of time to convince him.

"I'll go first," Amanda said.

Balancing with one foot on the big flat rock near the bank, she lowered her other bare foot toward the cool river water. Florencio's eyes were tortillas as he watched. He panted from fear. Would he have to carry his sister home if her feet turned to fins? How could they ever explain what they'd done?

Amanda pulled her foot out of the river, and water dripped from her toes. They examined her foot from toe to heel, poking it and looking for signs of metamorphosis.

No fin. No scales. They sighed in relief.

"You try, Florencio!"

"No, this is dangerous!" Florencio said, his chest heaving and nostrils flaring.

Florencio took a deep breath and put his toe in the water but didn't leave it in as long as Amanda did. The otherwise cool and refreshing water on Good Friday seemed like bubbling acid or some magical water that was forbidden to touch. He removed his toe from the water, and they examined his foot as well to notice any changes.

No fins. No scales.

Amanda took Florencio through the routine again. This time they stood with both feet in the flowing water. They both stepped off the banks of the river into the rocky river bottom with both feet sliding on the rocks and fully submerged. They looked through the rippling water; they still had feet. No fins. Why would adults lie to her?

Amanda picked up a wooden cup resting on a rock by the bank of the river. The wooden cup was typically used for pouring water when bathing by the river, but for Florencio and Amanda the wooden cup was a trap for tiny fish.

Amanda hiked up her dress and waded further, trapping fish and inviting Florencio to come deeper into the water. Their legs were covered. They decided one last time to come out of the water and check their legs for scales or tiny sprouting fins.

Amanda put down the wooden cup on the flat rock, now cooler from the dripping water from their suntanned legs. They looked at each other, smiled, took off their clothes and splashed into the water, laughing and playing. Amanda and Florencio went swimming on Good Friday, and grew no fins.

When Amanda and Florencio returned home, Amanda felt the urge to tell her mother that the story about the fish was not true. She rehearsed in her mind but never verbalized the conversation with her mother. The guilt would have shown through her like water sticking the gingham dress fabric to her skin after swimming. She pondered most of the day on these questions.

Amanda pushed open the large wood plank door of the adobe brick house her father had built less than a mile from the La Jigua town plaza. The house was quiet, so she slowed down and walked gingerly down the hallway as the late afternoon sunshine penetrated the house with bands of light coming through the openings where the brightly painted shutters had been pushed back on their hinges.

Florencio, Sr. had built a room in the house for his wife, Maria Antonia, so she could give birth to their children there. Maria Antonia prayed in the room every day and the children called it "Mama's Room."

No one except Maria Antonia was allowed to enter the room. When she needed help delivering or cutting the umbilical cord, Florencio, Sr. would enter the room to assist.

The door to the room was cut so the bottom half could be closed and little ones kept out when Maria Antonia needed rest or prayer. With the top half open, she looked out and talked to the older children and gave them instructions, and family members checked on Maria Antonia without entering the room. The older Madrid girls kept the red-orange floor freshly washed and shiny. Cleaning the floor was their only excuse to enter Mama's room.

Amanda could barely see over the half door but pulled herself with her hands on the top of it and raised herself just off her toes to see inside. She saw her mother praying. Amanda wanted to nestle into her lap as she prayed there with her hands on her face, sitting on the bed where she had given birth to so many babies. At times she would sleep in the room for several days before and after she gave birth.

Maria Antonia said from the day she gave birth to Amanda in 1957, she thought she looked like a *muñeca* doll, perfectly beautiful. Amanda Madrid was the sixth and middle child of eleven Madrid children. She didn't feel she belonged to the older group of five, with José away in El Salvador in high school, Fredy working on the farm, and Elsita like another mother to her. Instead, Amanda championed the younger group of five children and challenged the ideas and habits of the older group of five.

Compared to Maria Antonia's upbringing, Amanda's stable home with siblings and parents felt secure—like one of the nests she and Florencio, Jr. found in the crook of a tree. When Maria

Antonia was less than a year old, her mother attempted suicide by shooting herself with a gun. Responding to the report of the gunshot, a neighbor found her still conscious.

Stanching blood from the wound, her neighbor asked, "Why would you want to leave your baby girl without a mother?"

Perhaps the neighbor didn't expect an answer, but Maria Antonia's mother spoke.

"I have asked God," Maria Antonia's mother said, breathing between each word, "to take care of my baby the same way God took care of me when I was a girl."

Maria Antonia's mother lived a few hours but lost blood and consciousness, then died. Those last words of her biological mother were fulfilled in Maria Antonia's godfather and his wife, who took in baby Maria Antonia as their own. The biological father took no responsibility. The stepmother treated baby Maria Antonia with affection, as she did her biological children, but as Maria Antonia grew old enough to work, her stepmother treated her more like a family servant than a daughter. Then as a teenager, Maria Antonia met Florencio, and she escaped into marriage.

Hearing the stories of both her maternal grandmother's and her mother's abandonment planted seeds of compassion for orphans in Amanda's heart from a young age. When Amanda passed the birthing room in the hallway, she often felt the mysterious solace of the place where Maria Antonia fled after an argument with Florencio, Sr. or where she retreated in the mornings before others woke. Something magnetic pulled young Amanda toward "Mama's Room." If she could finally enter, breathe the air, run her fingers across the blanket on the bed, say a prayer, then all this would bring Amanda the same peace she saw her mother find there.

Amanda often watched her perturbed mother enter the prayer room and emerge later as the peaceful Maria Antonia again.

Amanda loved the prayer room and wanted to go there, but it was off limits.

One day Amanda couldn't breathe and it scared her. She had bronchial blockage from ascaris worms that seek to penetrate the lining of the lungs. Worms found their way to her nasal passage, blocking it. Amanda feared she would die. Sensing her fear, Maria Antonia carried Amanda to the prayer room to care for her in the bed where all but one of the Madrid babies were born. Maria Antonia curled around Amanda and whispered, *"Muñeca* doll, God loves you. He will heal you."

Amanda felt secure in the prayer room with her mother, and the fear of death subsided. A chamber pot by the door allowed Amanda to relieve herself of diarrhea, resulting from the worms, rather than venturing repeatedly to the outhouse in the dark.

Maria Antonia continued praying for Amanda. She placed her hands on Amanda's head and said, *"Gracias, Padre, por sanar a mi hija.* Thank you, Father, for healing my daughter."

Her mother's touch and prayers comforted Amanda when she felt as if she were going to die. Finally, after a long night, Maria Antonia extracted the worm, then Amanda breathed freely. She fell asleep as streams of morning sunlight reflected off the shiny red-orange tile floor.

Amanda often witnessed her mother comforting her siblings and neighbors this way. Particularly when Maria Antonia prayed over townspeople, she would say, *"Yo sé que mi Dios no me va a avergonzar.* I know that my God is not going to embarrass me." Amanda had always wondered what she meant by that. Why would God embarrass Maria Antonia?

Though she believed in God's healing, Maria Antonia also called the doctor in medical emergencies. Making a house visit, the doctor brought his leather bag with physician's instruments and supplies. Ordinary children saw a doctor's bag full of toys:

stethoscope, thermometer, medicines, reflex hammer, flashlight, tongue depressor. Amanda saw something different. She was attracted to the doctor, not because of his "toys" but because the doctor helped people.

From the moment she first saw the doctor helping her family, Amanda began thinking of becoming a doctor someday so she could help people. Her thoughts of becoming a *doctora* started as a fantasy she told no one about for many years. She knew of no female doctors, but at her young age neither did she know the obstacles in society to a woman becoming a doctor. But she knew instinctively that performing well in school was essential to fulfill her dream.

Amanda and her siblings walked one mile from their house, a modest adobe brick home with red clay roof tiles, to the school in La Jigua, directly across the tree-shaded plaza from the cathedral. Inside the building were several classrooms and each had children who spanned several grade levels.

Amanda started school a week late. The newest and youngest student in the class, Amanda could neither read nor write numbers higher than nine. She felt behind and wanted to catch up to the level of other children who could read and write. She bit her lip, held in the tears, and wiped her sweaty palms on her dress.

Making matters worse for Amanda, the teacher divided the class into two groups. Though the teacher didn't use the labels, it seemed to Amanda that "good" students composed group one and "bad" students composed group two. In order to be in the good student group, Amanda was required to write her numbers by tens. Could she do that now?

Amanda's heart beat like the heart of a bird with a broken wing she once held in her hands. She took short breaths, held back tears. She didn't want to be placed in the bad group, and she feared that if she failed this first assignment, the bad group was exactly where she was going. If that happened she might stay there the rest of the year, and the teacher might always view her as a bad student. Could she ask for help? If she asked for help, her teacher would immediately think her a bad student, even before she had a chance to write her numbers. So she raised her hand and asked to be excused to the toilet.

With the teacher's permission, she hurried out of the school building backdoor, down the steps and across the dusty playground behind the school to the outdoor toilet. Amanda went inside the small outhouse and latched the door. Her back to the wall, she squatted down but not to use the toilet. She just didn't know what else to do—she had to escape and be alone.

*"Padre, por favor ayúdame.* Father, please help me," Amanda said.

*"Quiero ser una buena estudiante.* I want to be a good student."

*"Si tu me ayudas voy a ser Cristiana el resto de mi vida.* If you help me I will be a Christian the rest of my life," she said aloud.

She exhaled and anxiety drained out. In place of worry, she felt peace. Earnest and sincere, Amanda opened her heart to God. She got up, unlatched the door, and walked back to the classroom, her chin no longer trembling. Coming out of the makeshift prayer room, Amanda imagined herself like Maria Antonia, more serene yet alert.

Though confident that God would help her, she still didn't know how to write by tens. When she returned to her table, she asked the tall boy sitting next to her—who she thought was very kind and sweet—for help writing numbers.

"I only know how to write my numbers from one to nine but can't write them by tens," Amanda said.

"Can you say, ten, twenty, thirty, forty, fifty?" the older boy asked.

Amanda repeated the numbers perfectly.

"Now write the number one, add a zero next to it. Write the number two, write a zero next to it," the boy concluded.

Amanda thought the boy explained how to write numbers in an unforgettably smart way. She picked up her pencil and wrote the numbers by tens with ease. She was proud of herself but also believed God sent the boy in response to her prayer.

When the teacher walked around the classroom checking the papers, she picked up Amanda's and said to the whole class, "Wow, look at this! She did not even have explanation."

Amanda smiled. She felt a new sense of power from prayer and writing her numbers. With the ability to write and understand numbers beyond nine, Amanda qualified as a courier to accurately bring required supplies from the *pulperia* (grocery).

One day at the *pulperia,* Amanda saw a man in the store with a bag of seeds. She noticed the transaction was not the normal direction. Instead of receiving money from a customer, the owner paid the man six cents a pound for the squash seeds. When she saw the money in the man's hand, she thought, *I can make money out of seeds? We feed the horses squash. I will pick up the squash seeds, dry them, and bring a bag to sell.*

When Amanda returned home, she began picking through squash that the horses had left after having their fill. Amanda's eldest brother saw her with a handful of seeds.

"What are you doing?" he asked Amanda.

"I'm not telling you," Amanda said.

"Why?"

"It's a secret," Amanda said, continuing to sort seeds.

Her brother shrugged and walked away. Amanda laid out the seeds on an old newspaper to dry in the sun. Then a few days later Amanda took a bag of seeds to the store owner, and he paid her six cents a pound. This was the first time she'd ever been paid money, and she liked it more than the candies the store owner gave her.

Near the end of her first day of school, when Amanda learned to write her numbers, she asked to be excused from class again. Returning to the outhouse and closing the door, she squatted down as she did earlier in the day.

Now she better understood what Maria Antonia meant when she prayed "*Yo sé que mi Dios no me va a avergonzar.* I know that my God is not going to embarrass me." Now Amanda believed: God helped her. He did not let her be embarrassed that day.

"*Gracias, Padre! Gracias! Me ayudaste! Voy a ser cristiana toda mi vida.* Thank you, Father! Thank you! You helped me! I'll be a Christian for the rest of my life."

Amanda believed in Maria Antonia's prayer, but she still wondered, *Who was right? Her mother who told her not to swim on Good Friday or her father who rode on the back of Jesus?*

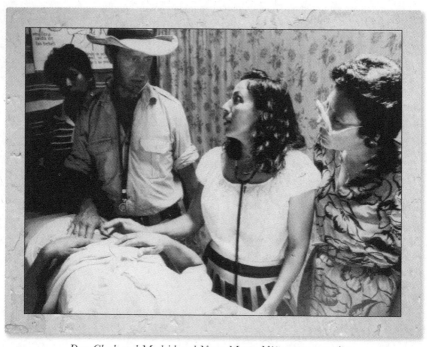

*Drs. Clark and Madrid and Nurse Marta Núñez treat a patient.*

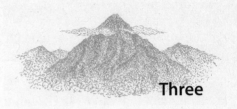

# Three

# ANYWHERE BUT THE WILD WEST

**In 1985, Amanda met a North American family relocating to Honduras.** *La Escuela Biblica* **(The Bible School) in Catacamas had asked Dr. Robert Clark and his wife, Doris,** to train Bible students with basic health care skills. The idea was that Bible students already dispersing throughout Honduras as preachers could also train in basic health care in order to benefit those communities with healing of soul and body.

The Clarks asked school officials if they knew anyone in the medical profession they could contact to learn what they needed to know about medical practices and needs in Honduras. The Bible School director gave the Clarks Amanda's contact information. When the Clarks traveled on their survey of Honduras to consider which city they would live in, they came to the capital, Tegucigalpa, where Amanda was completing medical school.

The Clarks contacted Amanda, who was intrigued to take a call from a North American physician. The Clarks asked if they could meet face to face to talk about practicing medicine in Honduras. Amanda suggested they meet at a pizza place on Morazan Boulevard in Tegucigalpa.

Tegucigalpa is nestled inside a series of bowls created by rings of mountains where the population lives perched—or so it seems from a distance—house upon house on bowl walls. Most people live on the sides of the bowl but do business, go to school, and attend church in the flat bottom of the bowl where government and commercial interests inhabit more valuable land.

Though she'd never met the Clarks, Amanda could pick them out easily at the restaurant. Even in a large city, in throngs of people on the streets or in the marketplace, the Clarks could not blend in. The shared family trait of blond hair caused Dr. Robert and Doris Clark and their two children to stand out in the crowd among Hondurans mostly with olive skin and brown hair. Hondurans might see the Clarks and assume they were tourists, flying in to the airport in Tegucigalpa but heading to the mountains, the beaches, or Mayan ruins. But the Clarks had other plans.

The Clarks were from Decatur, Georgia, and they had located in Guatemala but had been forced out during a civil war. Their motivation for meeting Amanda was not only to learn about medicine in Honduras but also to find someone like Amanda to work with in Catacamas. Under national law, no foreign doctor could work independently without the involvement of a Honduran doctor. Dr. Clark needed Amanda—when she completed her boards and became a certified doctor—in order to practice medicine legally in Honduras.

They exchanged greetings at the restaurant and sat down at a table. They ordered, drank sodas in slender glass bottles, and began talking about the mission in Catacamas. The Clarks described their plans for training health workers in the state of Olancho. Of the eighteen states in Honduras, Olancho got the nickname, "Wild West," not because it's directionally west in Honduras but for its characteristically "western style" of cattle raising, horse riding, and machetes carried like six-shooters attached to men's belts. And the "wild" moniker came from the lack of paved roads, electricity, medical care, and law enforcement.

A waitress brought their pizza, Dr. Clark said a prayer for their meal, and they ate. Doris cut her pizza with a fork, ate gingerly, and talked much less than Dr. Clark. She looked like Grace Kelly in jungle boots. Amanda couldn't believe a beautiful and proper woman like Doris would go to a place like Olancho. Amanda, on the other hand, had no intentions of moving to Olancho to practice medicine.

Amanda was interested, instead, in drug and alcohol addiction treatment in Tegucigalpa, not training medical volunteers in remote Olancho. She hadn't planned to even mention her experience in drug and alcohol treatment to the Clarks, because she couldn't imagine how missionaries would be interested in traveling from North America to Honduras in order to help alcoholics. She had no intention of telling them over this meal that she had felt a calling from God because of an experience with one patient during her emergency room rotation as a medical resident.

After eight years of university, medical school, and board tests at *La Universidad Nacional Autónoma de Honduras*, Dr. Madrid continued as a resident and military medical officer in the teaching hospital, a complex of fairly new medium rise buildings.

A man came into the ER, bleeding from deep cuts on his neck and arms. The attending doctor assigned Dr. Madrid to sew up the man's wounds. As she took the injured man's history, Dr. Madrid noticed his eyes were bloodshot and he blinked slowly. She got his name: Pedro. She asked how the cuts occurred, and he replied with slurred words. "I was mugged and knifed," the man said.

Dr. Madrid wrote what he said on his exam sheet. Then she wrote a question mark next to the part about being mugged. Plausible but questionable. His breath and sweat stank of beer. The location and types of cuts signaled something different to Dr. Madrid. She put down her clipboard then prepared the suture needle to stitch his wounds. With the man's arms laid out in front of her, she could see superficial wounds and scarring. She sutured and thought about what she wanted to say to her patient.

Perhaps she was moving more slowly because of her thoughts, because the attending physician walked by and said, "Hurry up, get that drunk guy out of here. We have patients who are truly sick and need to be seen."

Truly sick? This man has cuts all over his arms and neck, and he could be an alcoholic. He's not truly a patient who needs to be seen? She wondered if he needed psychological evaluation as well. As she sutured, she thought, *The reasons people take their own lives must be very powerful.* She had never understood why her maternal grandmother had committed suicide when Maria Antonia was only nine months old.

Like most medical residents, Dr. Madrid took pride in her suturing skills, but sewing Pedro's arms evoked only a feeling of futility. Merely stitching him up to "get him out of here" felt inconsequential to Dr. Madrid, like trying to block the sun with her finger.

"Pedro, why do you want to take your life away? What hurts so much that you don't want to live?" Dr. Madrid asked as she finished the last suture.

His eyes opened a little wider, he stared at the doctor, and his mouth opened but seemed unable to form any words. Then his face contorted and tears streamed from his drooping eyes.

ANYWHERE BUT THE WILD WEST

"My life is not worth living. I'm a nuisance to my family. It's better if I died. I only cause problems. My brothers, my family—they are decent people."

The attending doctor returned to call Dr. Madrid into the hallway.

"Doctor, I don't want to see you with that drunk guy one more minute. There are more patients to be seen," the attending doctor said.

"This patient—" Dr. Madrid said, pointing to her notes on the chart, "I think he has a suicidal intent—that's a medical emergency anywhere in the world. What should I do with him?"

"Let him go. He will most likely go back to the bar, get drunk, then his stitches will serve him nothing," the attending doctor said, and walked away.

The words, "his stitches will serve him nothing," jolted Dr. Madrid. She stood in the hallway physically hurting, feeling helpless, angry even, that she could not help Pedro more.

Walking back to the exam room, Dr. Madrid wondered why medical professionals like her attending doctor were so cynical. When she entered the room, she saw Pedro's wife. She was about thirty years old, much younger than Pedro, who was nearly fifty but looked older because of his condition. His wife was attractive, pregnant, and she held the hands of two young children.

Against her attending doctor's wishes and without his knowledge, Dr. Madrid took Pedro, his pregnant wife, and two children into an empty nearby room.

"Wait here," Dr. Madrid told Pedro and his family, and I'll come back soon. She reported back to her assigned room to take more patients, but between patients she returned to talk with Pedro and his family.

"How is your life at home?" Dr. Madrid asked Pedro's wife.

Pedro's wife hesitated, then started to cry.

"We suffer because of Pedro's drinking," she said. "He's promised many times to stop drinking, but he breaks his promises."

Pedro's wife still blamed herself, thinking somehow the fault was hers for all their problems. The children sat listening, tears welling up in their eyes. They could not have understood the depth of what was happening, only that both of their parents were crying.

Dr. Madrid left the room to make phone calls at the doctor's station. Where could she send Pedro? A detox unit? Addiction treatment center? She called other physicians and learned that the only option for someone in Pedro's condition would be the psychiatric hospital, Santa Rosita. She wrote a referral to Santa Rosita, medically discharged Pedro, but her unofficial discharge was a prayer for Pedro and his family.

After she watched Pedro, his pregnant wife, and two children walk away, Dr. Madrid wiped tears from her eyes, then sat down for a moment to compose herself. She closed her eyes and prayed: *With all my heart, Father, I want to make a way for people like Pedro—and his wife and children—to find hope, to restore their lives.*

By the time she met the Clarks for the first time at the pizza place, God was helping Dr. Madrid make that prayer a reality. She was helping to lead an effort to establish addiction treatment protocols for the Honduran military. With the help of Dr. Octavio Sanchez, a psychiatrist, Dr. Madrid traveled to the National Institute of Alcoholism in San José, Costa Rica, and under Dr. Sanchez she wrote a dissertation about addiction treatment. But she didn't tell the Clarks about any of that. She didn't think they would be interested.

The pizza was eaten and plates taken away, and Dr. Clark continued telling what he had planned for Olancho. Dr. Madrid was drawn to Dr. Clark's affable personality. He seemed adventurous, easy going, and she imagined him being fun to work with. He seemed to Dr. Madrid to be a good doctor who really wanted to help people—the very thing she wanted to do. She respected the Clarks' simple, sustainable idea: train preachers already traveling to visit villages in the mountains of Olancho so they could offer basic health services for people who have none. She had continued praying for wisdom about how to use her medical career to serve God, specifically in alcohol abuse treatment, somewhere in Honduras, just not Olancho. Not Catacamas. She feared a visit would send the wrong signal to the Clarks, that she was remotely interested in moving to Catacamas.

When Dr. Clark asked Dr. Madrid directly if she would like to move to Catacamas to work with their medical program, she didn't tell them about her work with addictions. Instead, Dr. Madrid told them the most compelling reason she felt committed to staying in Tegucigalpa: she didn't want to leave her sister.

Dr. Madrid's oldest sister, Elsita, was like a second mother to her. She cheered for Amanda to finish her residency and sewed clothes for her. Sharing an apartment in Tegucigalpa, they were not only sisters but also best friends.

One day Elsita pointed to lumps on her neck and asked Amanda what she thought they were. When Amanda felt the lumps in her sister's neck, she was startled, but she kept calm, not wanting to alarm her sister. After a full exam of her neck and throat, Amanda concluded that her sister would need a biopsy. Privately, Amanda prayed that God would take away the swelling miraculously, like Maria Antonia prayed so many times for people in Copán. She prayed that somehow she could trade places with Elsita. An appointment was made for a lymph node biopsy, and Elsita went to the hospital for the procedure. A few days passed while they awaited the results from the lab, and Amanda was the first to review them.

When she saw her sister's lab sheet, the faces of cancer patients Dr. Madrid had treated flashed through her mind, and her body trembled with fear and dread, because she knew survival with this type of cancer was rare. She couldn't imagine her sister like those patients, emaciated and sick to the marrow of their bones. Cancer treatments with good outcomes were rare in Honduras at the time.

So Dr. Madrid's motive for meeting with the Clarks was to confirm which hospital in the United States was best for cancer treatment, so she could take Elsita there. Dr. Clark affirmed what Dr. Madrid had already researched: MD Anderson in Houston would be the best and closest hospital in the United States for cancer treatment.

The Clarks understood that Dr. Madrid wanted to stay in Tegucigalpa close to Elsita, not four hours away in Catacamas. They left the restaurant where they had spent several hours talking, and they all resolved to pray for one another's challenges. The Clarks pressed Dr. Madrid to at least visit Catacamas after the Clarks located there a few months later, and Dr. Madrid said she'd think about it. That was the best she could offer, since she was intently focused on Elsita's treatment.

What possible good would a visit serve? She knew fairly well God had no plans for her in a place like Olancho. She had grown accustomed to the city life, and she didn't want to go to the wild and rugged mountain region of central Honduras. She'd never been to the Honduran state of Olancho where Catacamas was located, two hundred kilometers east of Tegucigalpa and as many clicks away from civilization, as far as Dr. Madrid was concerned. All she knew was that Olancho was the end of the road in eastern Honduras, a rough and tumble, poverty-stricken region she wanted nothing to do with. She wondered what her doctor colleagues would think. She flushed with embarrassment to think about telling them she was visiting such a place, much less moving there. How could she even mention this possibility to them? Plus, she had trained to be a doctor, not a trainer of volunteer health workers. She was equipped to treat patients, not teach. And in Olancho? No way.

Months after they had met in the pizza parlor in Tegucigalpa, Doris Clark called Dr. Madrid. The Clarks had made the move and were settling into life in Catacamas, getting ready to train healthcare workers and setting up a health clinic. Would Dr. Madrid like to come visit them and see what they are doing? Doris ended the call saying she was praying for Dr. Madrid's decision and believed God would show her what to do.

Amanda told her brother, Jesús, that Doris called. After hearing Amanda's excuses, Jesús said, "If you've been praying and a missionary calls you, don't you think it could be an answer to those prayers?"

Amanda did not argue with her brother but was arguing with God. *I don't want to go to Olancho! I know I told you I would go where you lead me, do whatever you call me to do. God, please, don't send me to Olancho!*

"Why don't you at least make a visit, then you will know better if it's truly the will of God," Jesús said.

"I'll think about it." In addition to listening for God's voice in the matter, Amanda heard the audible and competing human voices pulling her in different directions: Elsita, Maria Antonia, the Clarks, her medical colleagues, her brothers, the army calling on her to stay and serve. Visit the Clarks? Why?

A week later, in prayer she sensed God urging her with these words: *Go see the missionaries.* She did not hear or sense the words, "move to Olancho." Good! Just a visit. Her younger sister, Dina, asked if she could keep her company on the trip, and they drove from Tegucigalpa to Catacamas.

On the four-hour drive through mountains and fertile farm-land, Amanda bargained with God. *Just a visit! You know my dream, God. You placed it on my heart the night I treated Pedro! I want to start an alcohol treatment center. I don't want to move to Olancho!*

On the trip, Amanda discussed with her sister the offer she'd received from Standard Fruit Company in La Ceiba, where her mother and father and many siblings still lived with their families. How ideal to start an alcohol treatment center there among thousands of banana harvesters who needed help for themselves and their families suffering from alcoholism and abuse!

She resolved on the drive to Catacamas to tell the Clarks clearly that this was her plan—to start an addiction treatment center; she was sure they would simply back down from their offer to work together, that the goals were just too far apart.

Dr. Madrid and Dina arrived at the Clarks' home in Catacamas. Amanda smiled and hugged their two teenagers, Kendra and Robert Jr., who had grown since she saw them in Tegucigalpa, and the two sisters met other missionaries working with the Clarks.

Doris invited Amanda and her sister to relax after their long drive, and she brought them coffee. Amanda wrestled with what to say about her plans. She knew they would again ask her if she wanted to move to Olancho, but God seemed to be pulling her strongly in the direction of addiction treatment. How could her plans and the Clarks' plans be compatible? Why would the Clarks come all this way to establish treatment centers for addicts when worthy and innocent children, pregnant women, nursing mothers, and hard working men and women needed medical attention? They had come to train healthcare workers, not treat addicts. She had mixed emotions about this as well. Were addicts worthy of such expense and attention when they had made such terrible choices? Perhaps many people thought about addictions like her attending physician in the ER—move on to the worthy patients! Could that be a reason no one had ever established a rehab center for addicts in Honduras?

Finally the time came in the conversation when she was on the spot. The Clarks again told Amanda they'd been praying for her, for God to show her his will for her next step.

"As you've prayed, what has God shown you about coming to Olancho?" Dr. Clark asked.

"I've have been thinking and praying about this a lot. What you are doing is a great idea, to train preachers to do basic health care and to open a clinic here. I'm having a real struggle about this because what I really want to do is open a treatment center for alcoholics," Dr. Madrid said, and she watched the doctor's eyes for a reaction of disappointment.

Dr. Clark sat up straighter, leaned in. "Do you know how to treat alcoholics?"

"Yes," Dr. Madrid told him, "But I want to learn more, and I wanted to find out what they are doing in the United States. I know you—"

"Wait! Even in the United States few doctors know how to treat alcoholics!" Dr. Clark said. "But you know what? That's my dream too!"

Dr. Madrid was shocked. She wasn't expecting Dr. Clark to be interested in the least. And she'd convinced herself that his lack of interest in drug and alcohol treatment was one of the big reasons she could not move here. Now, her big excuse not to move to Olancho floated away. In a way, she had hoped the drug and alcohol treatment center would be out of the question and she could go forward with the idea in La Ceiba.

But now they had a common interest. The rest of the evening the Clarks and Dr. Madrid talked about drug and alcohol addiction treatment. She told Dr. Clark about Pedro, how God had planted an idea in her heart through one patient and his family who were suffering. She told him how she'd stitched him up but that sutures weren't enough, how she referred him to a detox and psychiatric hospital, but when she checked back a few days later she discovered the family had never arrived or registered. She was disappointed because Pedro had said during the exam that night in the ER that he would not fail again in his next attempt to kill himself. She wondered if he'd finally committed suicide and his wife had moved back in with her family.

Dr. Madrid told Dr. Clark that after seeing Pedro and his family, she resolved to do something more than stitching and referring: to establish new protocols for admitting, detoxing, and treating addicts and their families long-term. She told the Clarks how Pedro, his pregnant wife, and his crying children had broken her heart—and re-directed her career.

After hearing about Dr. Madrid's calling to addiction treatment, Dr. Clark had a revelation of his own.

"I'm a recovering alcoholic," Dr. Clark said.

Dr. Madrid, though initially stunned, thought about her physician colleagues—some did not believe themselves to be addicts, but they showed many of the signs. Dr. Clark's vulnerability touched another nerve in Amanda—she'd prayed to be useful and helpful to God and others since she was a little girl. Now the dual mission of telling about Jesus's love and healing people cut through her fear with a sharp scalpel, splitting her heart open. The mission of Christ poured in. God would not let her be embarrassed.

For the first time, she seriously considered moving to Olancho. Amanda needed a dream that fit her idealism and justified going to Olancho. Dr. Clark had delivered that. He said he would focus on training health care workers, but Dr. Madrid could focus on establishing an addiction treatment center.

When Dr. Madrid and her younger sister left the house the next day, Amanda felt as if she'd unloaded one burden and hoisted another onto her shoulders. She believed in the mission of preaching and healing, but why in Olancho?

Why couldn't it be anywhere but the Wild West of Olancho?

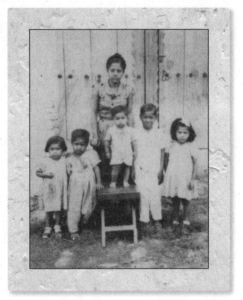

*Maria Antonia with five of her children.*

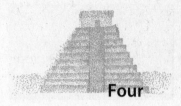

# Four

# MAYAN PRINCESS

**When Amanda returned from the** *pulperia* **(grocery) in La Jigua with a few coins from selling squash seeds, she found Florencio, Jr., and they walked up the white lime-**stone road to their grandmother Tula's and grandfather Gregorio's large adobe house. Tula and Gregorio Madrid's was the most distinctive house in La Jigua, on the highest hill on the family land.

In the large living and dining room, Tula had antiques and elegant furniture, and the breezeway in the center of the house was a plaza where the Madrid sons congregated before and after work to drink coffee and discuss the day's events. The floor was brick tile and over it, attached from the heavy exposed beams, hung several hammocks. Wrapped in the colorful woven fabric of one of the hammocks, Amanda cocooned herself from the chaos of living in the middle of eleven siblings, while Florencio, Jr. looked up in the trees for bird's nests.

Amanda rested in the hammock and felt smart. Amanda had heard her *Abuela* Tula say in a testimony to their small Evangelical

67

congregation that her children were all, "*Vivos para el pisto.* They are all smart to make money." Amanda felt smart to make money from the squash seeds.

Soon Florencio, Jr. grew tired of playing alone and called out to Amanda, and she went outside to where he was, next to a large wooden door on the side of the house that led to a basement. No other house in Copán had a basement like Gregorio's and Tula's house.

"What's in there?" Florencio, Jr. said.

"Children are forbidden to go in," Amanda said, cutting her eyes to the side.

"Yes, but what's—"

Amanda jiggled the doorknob, expecting it to be locked, but it wasn't. Amanda looked at Florencio, then looked back at the knob. She turned it fully and pushed the door open, and the rusty hinges moaned. Amanda first, then Florencio, stepped into the musty space under the house, their eyes darting side to side, lest a snake or worse—a basement ghost—surprise them in the dim light.

Clay pots against the wall enticed them. Amanda had heard people hid money in clay pots and buried them, and it was also said that ghosts haunt those places to guard the money. They checked in the pots and were disappointed to find nothing inside.

Then they saw a wooden chest that looked like a coffin. By its concealed mystery, the dust-covered box required them to open it. Small flies swarmed around them in the dark as their eyes adjusted and their only light was coming from the doorway. They worked the latch and lifted the top slowly.

For children at the house of an *abuela* (grandmother), they had struck gold: inside the box were old clothes, including a wedding dress and a doll that had a pretty dress but no hair. They played dress-up with the clothes and played with the doll.

Amanda wanted the doll badly, but she knew taking it would be stealing. She could tell Tula and Gregorio she wanted the doll, but then they'd know she'd been in the forbidden basement. After playing for hours, they returned everything back to the box just as they found it, slightly less neatly folded, closed the lid, and left the basement as it was—having added their finger smudges to every dusty surface.

A few days later, Amanda decided to tell her grandfather a lie that she had been dreaming about a *muñeca* (doll), and that it was in the basement, maybe in a box. She wondered aloud to her grandfather if she ought to go into the basement to confirm whether or not there really was a *muñeca*. No, Amanda was told, you can't go in the basement. Gregorio said Tula would be angry if the grandchildren entered the basement.

A few days later, on another visit to Tula's house, Amanda found the bald *muñeca* with the pretty dress in a big room they often played in upstairs. She asked no questions and played with the doll.

Maria Antonia called Amanda her *Muñeca*, and Florencio, Sr. called her his Mayan Princess, because Amanda was born in the far southern reaches of what had been the ancient Mayan kingdom, near the famous *Copán Ruinas*. Amanda's grandfather Gregorio was short, light skinned, and round-faced—often distinctive features of Mayans.

The Mayan empire stretched from Central Mexico to *Copán Ruinas,* where one of the most famous archaeological sites of Mayan culture unearthed an elaborate acropolis that time and dirt has mostly covered so that the uppermost pyramid is like the top of an iceberg where most is unseen. In the basement remains a system of tunnels built for access to crypts of Mayan rulers. The last known ruler of the Copán region, *Yax Pasah*, meaning First Dawn, built a monument known as Altar Q that memorialized a line of sixteen hereditary kings with depictions of handing to the next leader the mantle of leadership.

Amanda's father, Florencio, Sr., was the fourth of six children of Tula Gertrudis Enamorado and Gregorio Madrid. The Madrid brothers ran cattle and grew tobacco and grains, but there was rivalry between the Madrid siblings and in-laws, and Maria Antonia knew she was fighting a losing battle against so many family members. How could the mantle of leadership be passed to these brothers so all would have enough land?

Maria Antonia looked at her eleven children and dozens of growing nieces and nephews, and she did not like her prospects of prosperity and the hope of making enough money on the small patch of land to put her children through university or trade schools.

Maria Antonia said to Florencio, "I think we're living in a communist society on this family land." She wanted to move far away. Maria Antonia's and Florencio's many discussions about land began in low tones and ended up in shrill voices, Florencio storming out of the house, and Maria Antonia padding into the prayer room.

During those days Maria Antonia spent a lot of time in her prayer and birthing room. She prayed and envisioned the future, and she had logic-defying aspirations for her children, that they would all be college-educated. The land was large enough now for all of Tula's boys, but what about all of Maria Antonia's eleven children and many nieces and nephews?

Already Maria Antonia thought one of the brothers was taking advantage of Florencio, Sr. If Tula was already taking one son's side over her husband's, what hope did she have for her children to inherit enough land? When Maria Antonia and her mother-in-law, Tula, were in the same room, Amanda noticed her mother grew tense and quiet, and often after they'd spent time together, Maria Antonia would steal away to her prayer room.

Through Amanda's eyes, *Abuela* Tula looked like a queen, her hair braided and long, a purse over her arm, and an umbrella opened above her for shade as she rode on her horse wherever she went. She rode sidesaddle in a dress and seated very straight in the hornless saddle decorated with etched silver buckles. One day after she rode home from La Jigua and tied up her horse, she was talking with someone in the kitchen of her house and Amanda was nearby. Amanda overheard Tula talking about how Maria Antonia selfishly wanted more land and was thinking of moving.

One of Amanda's cousins said, "Abuela, can't you see Amanda's listening to you right now?"

Tula stopped talking about Maria Antonia, turned toward Amanda and began complimenting Amanda about how pretty she was, how smart, but Amanda didn't take the compliments, because she was hurt and didn't like what her grandmother was saying about her mother.

After years of tension between Maria Antonia and Tula, Amanda's mother thought she had the answer to her prayers. A traveling salesman came through La Jigua from time to time. He wouldn't sell Maria Antonia things as much as he would allow her to use them for a span of time so she'd learn that she could not live without them and pay for the items later: a hand mixer, a tortilla flattener, a bottle of this or that.

Maria Antonia would pay the salesman when he'd come back to town the next time. One day Maria Antonia asked the traveling salesman to watch for good available real estate on the north coast of Honduras. The next time the salesman came, he told her about a good piece of farmland outside of La Ceiba on the north coast. When the salesman left and Florencio returned from tending the cattle, Maria Antonia began working on her husband once again, this time with news of land.

"I have prayed a lot about this," Maria Antonia told Florencio. "I want my children to be educated."

"You think I don't want that for our children?" Florencio, Sr. shot back.

"And how are we going to accomplish this with so many family members and so little land?" Maria Antonia asked Florencio.

"We need to trust God, Maria Antonia!"

"I do trust God! I trust also in cattle and land to pay the bills."

"We can buy land in Copán."

"I don't want my children to be farmers, Florencio. The price for land in La Ceiba is good. I heard of a Christian man who wants good people on the land." She relayed the size and location of the land just as the salesman had described it to her, a day's drive to the east on the north coast of Honduras.

"What about our family? How can we leave our home here?"

"I have put this in God's hands," Maria Antonia said.

When the family got wind of the rumblings, there was an assault on Florencio and Maria Antonia to stay. Florencio's brother, Octavio, said, "You have all those girls, and in the north they might become prostitutes." There were a lot of North American and European men exporting bananas in the north coast, and the place was known for corruption and immorality. This thought scared Maria Antonia, and the fear for her children was piled upon guilt the family laid on her.

Octavio had been talking with Maria Antonia and Florencio in the sitting room, and Amanda was listening in the next room, her ear pressed to the door. "You are separating the family," Octavio said. "Why? Because you are too ambitious and greedy. You don't know what you will find in the north with its bad reputation."

Maria Antonia had heard enough about her daughters becoming prostitutes. She went to the kitchen to clean up and get the children to bed. After everyone was settled, she went into the prayer room and fell on the bed and sobbed.

She stayed in her prayer room for hours that evening, pleading with God for a resolution and that Florencio would swim like a fish upstream against the strong family current. She prayed for her children and caretakers for their house. They did not want to sell their house on the Madrid family land, but who would take care of it? She'd already burned bridges with many relatives, so asking them to care for the house would be out of the question.

Over the next few weeks, the decision became clear to Maria Antonia and Florencio somewhere in the midst of prayer, argument, and discussions with family. They made their announcement to the family that they were leaving. Florencio knew Maria Antonia would not be happy in Copán. Maybe she would be happy in La Ceiba.

They decided to keep the house in Copán, and part of the family would stay. Six of the children would go; four of the children would stay. They had ten children at the time. The eleventh and final Madrid child, Dina, was born later. The house would be left intact with all the furniture, the bed and nightstand and lamp in the prayer room, because Maria Antonia wanted the children to feel nothing had changed. But Amanda felt that everything had changed.

To her parents there was important logic to the division. Fredy, 19, and Elsita, 17, the oldest boy and girl, would stay and act as guardian parents to two of the youngest who could handle themselves without their mother: Amanda, 9, and her next youngest brother, Florencio, Jr., 7.

The very youngest children, Elder, 5, Ana, 3, and Antonia, 1, would need to go with Maria Antonia to La Ceiba. Florencio,

Sr. would need capable workers on the farm outside La Ceiba, so they took Jesús, 11, Mery, 13, and José, 15. Education motivated Maria Antonia and Florencio as well. La Jigua had no high school, and the closest high school was in Santa Rosa, the capital city of the state of Copán. They reasoned that sending the children there would split the family anyway, so why not take them to new land and a high school in La Ceiba?

The day of the move was chaotic. Jesús and José packed in the big room for the boys; Mery packed in the room with the girls, including items for her younger sisters, Ana and Toñita. The bus would arrive soon, so they were rushing to include everything they intended to take to La Ceiba, which was two days journey distant on the north coast.

Elder, Ana, and Antonia were confused or oblivious to what was happening around them. One of Amanda's chores was caring for baby Antonia, changing her diapers, saving morsels of food to feed her. The family gave her the nickname, *Toñita*, Little Antonia. Amanda would gladly go along to care for Toñita if called upon by the family. Amanda held Toñita tightly, wishing and praying away this family split that broke two big places in her heart—the little girl's heart to be with Maria Antonia and the motherly heart for Toñita.

Neighbors gathered to say goodbye to Maria Antonia, Florencio, Sr., and the six children going with them. Tula and Gregorio walked down the hill from their house to say goodbye to their son and his family, to comfort Maria Antonia that they would watch out for the four children staying behind.

La Jigua, Copán was small enough that the driver of the 1950s model public transportation bus could meet most passengers in front of their houses if they had lots to carry. After getting a message in their bus reservation that the Madrid family was moving, that they'd have extra luggage, the driver had agreed to stop in front of Florencio's and Maria Antonia's house.

The pace turned frenetic as neighbors lifted suitcases up to the driver's helper on the top of the bus to be tied down. Amanda's chest tightened as she watched her siblings racing back and forth from the house to the bus. Was this really happening?

Amanda thought her mother would be emotional, but Maria Antonia remained stoic, saying goodbye to each of the children.

Seeing her mother's example, Amanda held back her tears— until she said goodbye to her younger sisters, Ana and Toñita. When baby Toñita reached out her hands to her former caretaker, tears rolled down Amanda's cheeks as the larger part of the family boarded the bus.

The bus engine revved and the driver jammed the gears. Exhaust poured out the back of the bus while neighbors stood in front of the Madrid home, watching a family rent in two by ambition, desire for land, and family conflict. The door unfolded and locked in place, and finally the bus roared away for the two-day trip through the industrial city, San Pedro Sula, and further east to the port city, La Ceiba.

The bus gained speed, and Amanda ran after it then stopped. She watched the bus disappear over the horizon, leaving only a cloud of dust. Tears streamed down her face like drops of rain flowing down Tula's umbrella.

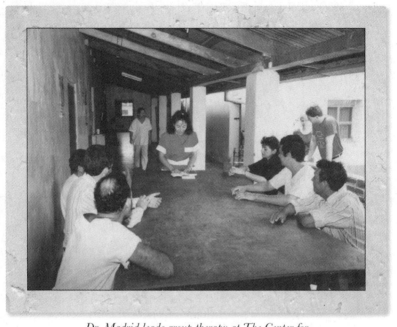

*Dr. Madrid leads group therapy at The Center for Rehabilitation for Patients with Addictions (CEREPA).*

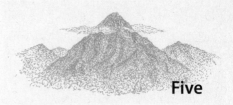

# Five

# A SOBERING PLACE

**One night, after visiting the Clarks in Catacamas, emotion filled Dr. Madrid as she wrestled with God in prayer. She prayed for God to change her heart from being embar-**rassed in the eyes of her medical colleagues to being proud she was going to Olancho. She wasn't proud, though. So she prayed Maria Antonia's prayer, *"Yo sé que mi Dios no me va a avergonzar.* I know that my God is not going to embarrass me." She prayed for her family to accept her calling, to support her move to the Wild West. Finally she declared to herself and to God, "Yes, this is what I'm going to do."

Reactions were mixed and she got strange looks from her Honduran medical colleagues when she told them she planned to move to Olancho, but she was not embarrassed. God had answered her prayer. After living in Tegucigalpa twelve years for university, medical school, and work as a military medical officer, Dr. Madrid moved to Catacamas in 1987.

Arriving to stay, not just to visit, in the poorly developed town of Catacamas unnerved Dr. Madrid. On the potholed streets mules pulled carts, children drove cattle, stray dogs barked, and trucks hauled fruit to the central market. Catacamas was built on the lower slope of a mountain where a twenty-foot cross placed at the summit seemed to watch over the town.

Though disgusted with the condition of the town, Dr. Madrid walked through Catacamas meeting people, discovering how glad they were to have a new doctor. She visited Alcoholics Anonymous meetings, telling groups about her plans to open a treatment center in her first year. She also traveled with Dr. Clark to mountain jungles, treating patients with acute illnesses, giving immunizations, treating for worms, and checking on pregnant women. Assisting the doctors were a healthcare trainer from Cuba named Ania Fernandez, a Honduran nurse named Marta Núñez, and other Hondurans and North Americans. Dr. Clark also brought his son, Robert, Jr., to the mountains with him. Dr. Madrid noticed Robert, Jr. seemed to enjoy being in the mountains more than being in school, and in many ways these trips with his father became his education during those formative adolescent years.

Both doctors were adventurers, so riding horses up the mountain posed no problem for them, and they enjoyed the slow pace of travel and the interaction with villagers along the way. The first time Dr. Madrid rode up the mountain with a medical team in a train of horses carrying medical staff and supplies, she treated dozens of patients with conditions such as measles, malaria, diarrhea, and machete cuts.

Machete cuts could be self-inflicted while chopping a vine, but most of the time men arriving for medical care with wounds had been fighting with machetes. One young man's arm, hands, and fingers were so deeply lacerated by machete cuts from another man in a quarrel, that Dr. Madrid suggested he travel back with them and go to the hospital. He refused, so the doctor did surgery in abysmal light with mosquitoes buzzing in their ears. Physician Assistant Katherine Evanson helped Dr. Madrid find the two ends of a tendon and sew them together. When Dr. Madrid sutured the wound closed, the man—awed that he could move his fingers—broke the stitches open by bending too forcefully. Dr. Madrid re-sutured the now oozing wounds and sent him home.

The medical crew slept that night in hammocks slung from the rafters at a local church. The next day Dr. Madrid saw the man again, and he could barely move his hand. Again, she urged her patient to return with them to the hospital, but he did not want to go. So Dr. Madrid immobilized the man's hand, gave him antibiotics, instructions for care of the wound, and physical therapy exercises after healing.

Weeks later, on another visit to the mountains, Dr. Madrid saw a man running toward their train of horses on the road.

"Dr. Madrid! Dr. Madrid!" It was the father of the young man she'd sewn up after a machete fight.

Dr. Madrid dismounted her horse and walked to the house where they saw that the young man's arm and fingers were healed. She removed his stitches and told him to continue the physical therapy she'd prescribed. Finally, they prayed and thanked God for the miracle.

One day a man came in to a mobile clinic complaining of an earache. Dr. Clark examined the man's ear canal with his otoscope, and it seemed a foreign object had gotten in his ear. Carefully Dr. Clark reached in with instruments to try to pull out the object without pushing it farther in. Marta Núñez helped steady the man and talked to him while the doctor did the extraction. When the object finally came out, Dr. Clark held it up, smiled, then laughed with relief that both doctor and patient felt. The object inside the patient's ear was a bumblebee. Unlike honeybees, bumblebee stingers do not have barbs, so the bumblebee can sting repeatedly. How many times had the man been stung inside his ear canal?

In another remote mountain village, a woman came to the clinic to talk about problems she was having with her pregnancy. Dr. Madrid heard the woman's history, examined her, and feared she might miscarry again. In times like this Dr. Madrid realized the intense need to train health care volunteers to discuss health and nutrition for families, particularly those with children and pregnant women.

"You are so anemic you may not be able to carry this baby to term." Dr. Madrid said. "And if you keep trying to carry babies in this condition, it's going to kill you."

Later in the day the woman's husband walked to the clinic to find out for himself what this female doctor dared to tell his wife—that she could not carry babies to term in her condition.

Dr. Madrid took the man aside and explained the dangers his wife faced in her anemic condition. She suggested ways he could take care of his wife and not treat her merely like a baby producer. For a source of protein, Dr. Madrid suggested he keep some of the eggs to feed his wife and young children, rather than selling them all. The man was so angry to be told what to do by a woman that he took a swing at Dr. Madrid. She ducked to avoid a slap on the face.

Just getting to the mountain villages was difficult, so being swiped at by patients was not an easy pill for Dr. Madrid to swallow. The crews eventually used vehicles to travel higher in the mountains, but roads were often impassable, and they would finish the journey on horseback—sometimes only after laboring for hours digging the vehicle out of the mud repeatedly. Creeks flowed over many mountain roads because no culverts passed underneath to allow water to pass. Medical crews in Predisan vehicles often forded streams, hoping the vehicle wouldn't float away with them inside. Dr. Madrid learned how to use a winch to pull the vehicle out of the mud.

On one of those mountain trips, a group had gone out to do vaccinations. At the time there was no bridge over the Cuyamel River. On the way up the mountain roads the river was passable. But in the days that passed, the river rose. When they reached the river on the return trip, they had to decide: cross the rising river in the Landcruiser or wait till the river receded.

A local Honduran man volunteered to attach the truck's winch cable to himself and wade out into the river to see how deep it was. Four feet deep, with swiftly flowing water. Don Gil, the driver, knew it was more than deep enough to sweep the vehicle away.

"What do you think we should do?" Dr. Madrid asked Don Gil.

"If I was alone, I would not pass over the water at this level. But if you tell me to do it, I will—in the name of Jesus." Don Gil said, trying to smile.

The group voted. Four wanted to go—mostly men—and the rest wanted to stay, mostly women.

The Toyota Landcruiser was equipped with a diesel engine and a high air intake mounted on its side. A diesel engine can be submerged and still run as long as the air intake is above the water—sort of like a snorkeler breathing through the pipe. The men were anxious to see if this really worked. The men reasoned, "Why would they make these high intakes if you don't use them?"

"If the water goes over the top of the intake," said Don Gil, "It's over."

At first some of the women wanted to stay on the shore to see if this worked. They could cross on a horse or wade across holding a guide rope strung across the river, but more weight would give the vehicle more traction, so they decided everyone should get in the vehicle and cross together.

"If the men drown, the women drown with you," one woman said.

The same man who had tested the waters earlier attached the winch to himself again, this time crossing completely and securing the winch cable around a large tree trunk on the opposite bank. The winch cable would be a lifeline if the water swept the vehicle down river—that is, if the cable didn't snap from the weight of the vehicle and force of the water. On the bank of the river, Don Gil shifted the vehicle into low four wheel drive then slowly entered the river so the tires would not swim but stay grounded on the river rocks.

When the Landcruiser entered the river, the water was so deep it rose to the top of the doors, and the passengers wondered aloud if the water would come in the windows. The car interior seemed to darken, no one could hear the engine, and everyone panicked, even Don Gil.

Strangely, however, the vehicle kept moving. The engine had not stopped. The water simply muted the engine sound. As they crossed the river, the group remained silent except for some groans from worried passengers. Would they get out? They prayed and called on Jesus—could he send Moses to part the waters?—to help get them across without the vehicle dumping sideways and emptying them all into the river or trapping them helplessly while the water poured in. Finally they emerged on the far bank and again heard the roar of the engine as it pulled the vehicle and the medical staff onto the riverbank.

Everyone cheered and clapped and hugged each other.

Because of these harrowing experiences, the health care teams often parked the vehicle, crossed the river holding a rope or cable, then rode horses to complete the journey up the mountain. Riding gave Drs. Madrid and Clark time to talk and strategize about their work and the future of clinics in the mountains. Well into the first year, the mobile clinics were succeeding in the mountains with local Hondurans loaning horses, manpower, and training to be health care workers in the clinics.

"Amanda," Dr. Clark said one day as they rode along under the shade of pines and large oaks on soft dirt and gravel roads, "you've worked hard since you arrived, preparing to open the addiction treatment center. I want you to know you can spend less time in the mountains so you'll have more time to focus on launching the center."

"What about the work in the mountains?" Dr. Madrid asked.

"Even if it means not coming to the mountains as much, I want you to be able to spend more time developing the addiction treatment center in Catacamas."

They decided she ought to rent a house to start the detox and treatment center. Feeling great, she challenged the doctor to a horserace. Making sure the pack horses were un-tied from hers and re-attached to the horses of other riders, she kicked her horse's sides, slacked the reigns, leaned forward and slapped the horse playfully and called out, "Ha!" She ran the horse for about a quarter mile, and when Dr. Clark finally caught up to her, he suggested she slow down, that she was riding too wildly.

"Wild" could describe what Doris Clark thought of Dr. Madrid's vision to build a new large building for the alcohol treatment center. When Dr. Madrid brought a printed list of the resources needed to build a center, Dr. Clark and U.S. medical systems consultant Justin Myrick were elated. Doris, however, was shocked at the daunting list.

"How are we going to do all this?" Doris asked.

The list looked insurmountable: rent a house for which there was no money, build on land they did not have, use heavy equipment they did not own, in order to accommodate and treat forty patients who had probably spent all their money on their addictions. The prospects for success looked bleak.

"What about beds, tables, and equipping a kitchen?" Doris asked.

Dr. Madrid had already identified a carpenter who could build beds.

"What about fundraising?"

"We'll travel to the United States and talk to churches there."

"What about staff? Who will pay them?" Doris asked.

Dr. Madrid told Doris and Dr. Clark her plan to apply for Peace Corps workers and for Honduran government mental health care workers—many of whom could be paid by government programs or grants. Dr. Madrid enlisted her friend, Eda Rivera, to organize the kitchen. She recruited nurses and administrative staff.

"How will you pay them?"

Dr. Madrid didn't have answers for all of Doris's admittedly important questions. Every dreamer needs a person grounded in reality to ask vital questions and press the dreamer to put steps to the plan, and that's exactly what Doris helped both doctors do. She would become the backbone of the organization, coordinating clinic activities and projects.

Meanwhile, Dr. Madrid worked in the Good Samaritan Clinic in the mornings and trained health care workers in the afternoons. Seeing her diligence, Dr. Clark agreed to help pay half the rent for a house to start the treatment center.

One day Amanda visited one of the medical field workers and thought her house would be perfect for the rehab center.

"Are you interested in renting your house?" Dr. Madrid asked the woman.

"No, my husband built it for me and my children. He passed away. This is our home."

Amanda really wanted that house. The configuration was perfect for a temporary rehab center as they prepared to build a permanent center. She went back to the widowed mother and explained the idea to her. She was moved by the idea, taking her family to a house next door and allowing Dr. Madrid to rent the house her husband completed shortly before his death.

Now they had a house but no patients.

Most mornings Dr. Madrid walked for exercise with health-care volunteer and best friend, Eda, who operated a hair salon at a corner shop in Catacamas. Early one morning while enjoying their routine of walking and gabbing, the two women saw a man near a cantina foraging for food in a putrid pile of garbage strewn on the ground. They figured him to be in his sixties. He looked old, thin, worn down by life, viciously drunk.

"We should talk to this man," Eda said. "Maybe he could come to the addiction treatment center."

They agreed to approach the man. When they walked toward him, the man took a step back, his head bobbing back and forth.

As soon as they could look into the man's eyes and ask him a few questions, they found out the man they figured to be at least sixty was really thirty-six years old. Substance abuse aged him in double time.

"Want to go to a place where you can get food and health care?" the doctor asked the man.

Unresponsive, he continued sifting through the trash.

Tiny worms crawled on his fingers and ears. He reeked of alcohol and urine.

What Eda and Amanda decided to do that day set a new course for the addiction treatment center. They got on either side of the man, each woman taking one of his arms, and escorted the man, named Victor, away from the trash heap, down the street, to the rented treatment house.

In an outdoor washroom they hosed him down and meticulously picked the worms off his hands and ears. They asked some neighbors for a pair of clean clothes for him. When a neighbor returned with the clothes, the man changed into the fresh pants and shirt.

Victor was the center's first resident patient. And this was a victory for the center to begin doing something with a patient and start developing the program, *El Centro de Rehabilitacion del Paciente Adicto,* The Center for Rehabilitation for Patients with Addictions (CEREPA).

In the following days, townspeople heard about Victor, knew he was one of the town drunks, and they were amazed that he could get sober. People in Catacamas began to see that a residential program for severe alcoholism could save the lives of many addicts. The word spread about CEREPA and others entered the program.

Jorge Yanez, who took care of shopping and other administrative activities at CEREPA, was the first person hired exclusively for the center. He graduated from a training program for health care workers. Since Jorge lived in Sosa, far from the city, Dr. Madrid offered him a room in the rented house. Marta Núñez, one of the trusted nurses who had been by Dr. Madrid's side in the mountain mobile clinics, worked in CEREPA as a therapy nurse.

As more addicts came, the house proved inadequate, and those who truly needed to stay escaped to find alcohol or drugs. So Dr. Madrid sought out Honduran and North American architects to sketch plans for a building that would house up to forty patients and prevent them from escaping. A committee of Hondurans and North Americans that had been formed to start CEREPA developed a rough sketch of a hacienda-style building with an enclosed plaza that would secure patients inside.

The committee saw the need for addiction treatment, wanted to act, but with no land, no money for materials, no builders, how could they?

The committee asked the Catacamas municipality for a piece of land, but the city rejected the request. Still, the committee persisted and reapplied to the municipality. After three applications submitted to the city, the mayor granted the land to build the center. The problem, however, was the city building permit gave them a very limited amount of time to build the structure.

They had to quickly raise funds and donations of materials. The committee called in every favor from friends they could imagine. A structural engineer named Mario Lobo and medical systems specialist Justin Myrick designed the building based on a center in Guatemala. The Honduran Olympic soccer team traveled to Catacamas to play a match to raise funds for CEREPA. Dr. Madrid and her roommate and co-worker, Katherine, sold their horse saddles in order to buy plane tickets to the United States, where they traveled to raise funds. Sunny Hills Church in Southern California was the first church to financially support CEREPA.

Catacamas Mayor Toño Salgado donated the use of heavy machinery and men to level the ground for the foundation of the facility. After the groundbreaking ceremony, which was attended by media and city officials, Dr. Madrid oversaw the building project. She jogged from her house to CEREPA early each morning to check on the progress and speak with the builder, Isaul Hernandez.

Together with the builders and designers, Dr. Madrid stretched the thousands of dollars initially raised, asking friends and neighbors for simple but expensive building materials like cement. Businesses donated five hundred bags of cement. In this way the building design, materials, and labor costs were kept low.

The CEREPA staff moved from the rented house to the building in 1990. Dr. Madrid wanted CEREPA to be self-sustaining. She didn't want to turn away patients due to the lack of resources. She wrote a proposal for Canadian government aid to establish a self-sustaining project. The project included a staff carpenter who would teach carpentry skills to residents. They would build furniture to sell in order to provide income for the center. Mennonites trained residents how to bake all kinds of bread to sell in the groceries around Catacamas.

They planted fruit trees, including oranges, lemons, and papayas. They planted a vegetable garden, raised rabbits, and stocked a fishpond.

As the months and years passed, the goals of those who managed the businesses and the goals of the therapists in the center clashed. Therapists needed long hours daily to work through patients' addictive behavior in group sessions. Those trying to produce products for sale needed manpower. Conflict arose between economic production and rehabilitation of patients. No one seemed able to resolve the dilemma. The businesses began to require more manpower to run than the center could provide. After all, the residents were required to stay in the center, not go into the marketplaces. They were afraid that patients who went out would find ways to get drugs or alcohol in those marketplaces. So the delivery of bakery goods and furniture to the markets relied on employees and therapists of the center.

The laborers were paid fair wages and the carpentry shop used legal wood. Competitors, meanwhile, often used illegally cut hardwoods and paid less than CEREPA, so it was difficult for the furniture project to compete on price. At the fish pond, meanwhile, problems were self-inflicted. Hungry neighbors caught and ate the fish before they could spawn enough to reproduce. CEREPA staff was not opposed to helping feed hungry friends, but they overharvested and depleted the fish. The guards were fed at the center but they also wanted to take additional food home to their families. On one occasion administrators interrupted a guard stealing chickens from the coop. The guard said, "I was just borrowing a hen to warm extra eggs at my house, but when the eggs hatch, I will bring the hen back." The theft wasn't the guard's first offense and he was fired.

One by one the businesses crashed from self-inflicted wounds, conflicts, and competition. The furniture shop and bakery closed, and the pond and chicken coop did not produce anything marketable. The upside was that the therapists now had all the time they needed with patients as a captive audience.

The demise of income generating projects, however, pressured Dr. Madrid and the Predisan board to come up with more money to continue running the center.

Though the majority of those treated for alcoholism and drug addiction were men, Dr. Madrid also treated women. When the center moved to the new facility, staff decided to reserve a room with several beds for women. The proximity of the men's and women's rooms became a problem when both men and women tried to break the lock to the door between them. Dr. Madrid realized that at the same time they were trying to help, they were also setting everyone up for bigger problems with attractions between men and women. The staff later modified the building so women had a separate wing, rather than only one room.

Over the years of Dr. Madrid's research and observations, she learned more about the differences in addiction treatment of men and women. She then trained the staff to understand these differences. Other organizations in Honduras have used the CEREPA model of treatment, but CEREPA has remained the only place in Catacamas for treatment of women with addictions.

Over the years CEREPA has treated four thousand patients for addictions by bringing them into the residential center.

Mario Hernandez was an alcoholic who entered the residential center but left before completing the program. He returned to alcohol and drugs. He abused his wife and beat his children when he was drunk. His brothers wanted to take him to another program, but they could not get him to agree to go. They finally compromised on bringing him back to CEREPA. Upon his return, he had hallucinations during his second detox, but he endured, became sober, and worked harder on his issues. The second time in CEREPA, Mario took responsibility for his own recovery, and asked for a family visit. The family came and joined some therapy sessions with Mario. Together the therapists, Mario's family, and Mario made a decision that he would stay longer than the required eight weeks—an additional four weeks—to continue working on his life issues.

When Mario returned home to his village in the mountains, he attended a local AA meeting in a nearby village, then started a meeting in his own village. Another man who Mario met at AA gave him a construction job. Later, he attended medical volunteer training at Predisan and qualified to work in one of the outpost clinics. After working a few years in the clinic, Mario was accepted into the university. To help put himself through school, he ran a chicken business. He continues to help other addicts in AA, particularly staying in touch with CEREPA to help former patients from the residential center assimilate back into their lives, to make new friends who are not addicts, and to stay away from the temptations to relapse.

Not everyone ended their program successfully. One patient was sent home after a visit from his girlfriend. The director, Karla Posantes, walked in when the couple was about to have sex in a guest visiting room. The man became violent and threw a printer at Karla. Mario was in the center at the time and heard the commotion and came to help Karla. The man threatened Karla and left the room in a rage. Karla started the process of talking with the girlfriend and family members, telling them their patient would have to leave if he could not calm down and behave within the standards of the center. He continued to make threats and was sent home, but he stayed in Catacamas and waited for Karla outside the fenced property and continued to threaten her from a distance. She called police and as they drove up the man fled and never returned to CEREPA.

A wealthy man named Fredy Garcia entered CEREPA so high on cocaine and inebriated from alcohol that he slept three days in the center. Fredy had made lots of money, and when one of his friends introduced him to cocaine, he bought two ounces a week and shared it with friends. In a few years he had squandered his money and property on his addiction. Weeks passed and he sobered but hardened against staff and became obstinate. Six weeks into treatment, Fredy finally accepted responsibility for his addiction. He participated willingly and productively in the final six weeks of the program.

CEREPA released Fredy after twelve weeks, but his problems continued when he returned to his life and tried to start a new business. His business associates had already been burned by his addiction. They didn't believe he had changed. But he was a different man. He started a small business without much help from others, and he multiplied his capacity with each success. Eventually he made enough money to build a house for his children who had disowned him during his downward slide. His wife didn't want to return to him, but Fredy still supported her financially. She needed to see Fredy prove his love by remaining sober a long time. After three years, the two re-married. Fredy has maintained sobriety and regularly sends both patients and donations to CEREPA.

Each year CEREPA staff honors graduates of the program with a party to celebrate their accomplishments together. With each graduate, Dr. Madrid sees evidence that her dream of establishing an addiction treatment center has come true. But the more she saw addiction in families, the more Dr. Madrid knew she had to attack the problem upstream, with children and teenagers. The staff developed an addiction prevention program, and thousands of youths have participated.

Perhaps those young Hondurans will never have to enter CEREPA like Fredy Garcia did. Fredy had a second chance, becoming like a child with a fresh start. He called CEREPA his "second womb," because it was there that he was born again.

Just as patients were finding hope, Dr. Madrid wondered how CEREPA and Predisan would survive after income-generating efforts failed, and the organization was about to lose one of its founders.

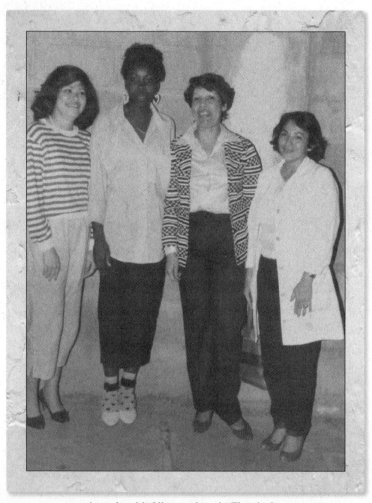

*Amanda with fellow students in Tegucigalpa.*

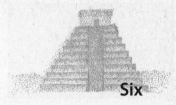

Six

# WORKING THE PROBLEM

**The morning after eight of her family members left La Jigua, Amanda opened her eyes, sat up in bed, and felt the sadness you feel when you dream someone you love** has died. The sun rose over the mountains to the east, roosters crowed, dogs barked, and birds chirped morning tunes in the treetops, but everything else, it seemed, had changed for Amanda.

She expected to see Maria Antonia praying in her sacred room. Where was the smell of coffee, warm tortillas, and *frijoles* wafting through the house? Maybe if she walked down the hallway to the dining room, Florencio, Sr. might be sitting at the kitchen table reading the Bible and drinking coffee, as always. Maria Antonia and Florencio, Sr. were not in their usual places. They were gone. No, this wasn't a nightmare she could end by waking up, by falling into the arms of her mama or papa. Amanda's heart felt empty, like the Madrid house.

To help the remaining children feel at home, Maria Antonia left the Madrid home furnishings, beds, and kitchen as they were

95

before the eight family members left. Her older sister, Elsita, older brother, Fredy, and her younger brother, Florencio, Jr. remained, but now she could see only empty chairs where her sisters Ana, Mery, and Toñita would be sitting.

Amanda dressed and went outside with her older sister, Elsita, and they built a fire in the cooking pit to make breakfast. After a trip to the outhouse, Amanda fetched water from the tank in a kettle, placed it over the fire to heat for coffee and bath water, and quietly the two girls rolled out a mixture of corn flour and water. They cooked corn tortillas and spread mashed beans on them. Amanda had set food aside for Toñita before she realized it wouldn't be necessary.

Fredy would wake up soon, wanting to bathe then eat, so the girls supplied both hot water for his bath and hot food for his stomach before he walked a mile to the school, where he was one of the teachers. In the new family arrangement, Fredy became Amanda's guardian at home as well as her teacher at school.

Amanda and Florencio, Jr. walked to school on the plaza in La Jigua. Elsita would often join them on the walk to school, but her workload caused her to spend some of her day managing the livestock, garden, shopping, and cooking for the family of four.

One day at school Fredy asked Amanda to come up to the blackboard to compete with her cousin in a math race. Amanda didn't want to compete with her cousin. She stared at the chalk in the tray but did not pick it up. Her cousin picked up a piece of chalk, raising his eyebrows as if to say, *Pick up the chalk, your brother's coming!* Instead of working the problem in a math race against her cousin, Amanda folded her arms and struck a stiff angled pose.

Fredy rose from his chair, walked toward Amanda, threatening with his eyes, gritting his teeth.

"*¡Escriba el problema, Amanda!* Work the problem, Amanda!" Fredy said.

Amanda remained silent. She raised and lowered her folded arms to emphasize she was not budging.

"*¡Obedeceme!* Obey me!" Fredy said through clenched teeth.

"No." Amanda turned away from Fredy toward the blackboard and froze.

"You better do this!" her brother said, giving a vague threat of punishment.

Amanda held her ground, not wanting to compete against her cousin. More than that, she wanted Fredy to know he could not control her.

Fredy led Amanda by the arm outside the classroom where he forced her to kneel down on pebbles that bit into the thin layer of skin over her knees like hundreds of dull needles. She panted quietly from the pain, squinted her eyes, and gritted her teeth. Amanda could only endure the pain for a minute before her body lurched forward, and she braced herself with her hands.

Fredy punished Amanda harshly at home as well. One day when Amanda resisted Fredy's authority, he poured coarse hardened cornmeal on the concrete floor and made Amanda kneel down on bare knees until she begged forgiveness. The pain was unbearable, like Fredy's tyranny over the home, and Amanda was too stubborn to beg forgiveness.

As the months passed, the relationship between Amanda and Fredy deteriorated further with Amanda's resentment and Fredy's tyrannical duties *in loco parentis*. One of Amanda's friends suggested Amanda do something that might free her from her misery.

"Write sad things in your letters to your mother," Amanda's friend told her.

"Why?"

"So your mother will feel sorry for you and come and get you."

A look of discovery came across Amanda's face and she said, "What if I write to my mother and say that I'm so sad that I want to die?"

"Good!" Amanda's friend said. "That will make her want to return and get you!"

"Yes, I think it will!"

Later, Amanda wrote her letter, saying she wanted to die, and she took the letter in a sealed envelope to her grandmother, Tula, who helped her mail it at the post office.

Time passed and Florencio, Sr. made one of his periodic visits to check on the four children, the land, and the cattle. Amanda's spirit soared when she heard the bus approaching. From a distance she saw her father get off the bus in town and walk up the road home. She called for Florencio, Jr. and the pair ran down the white gravel road to meet him. On a previous visit, Florencio, Sr. had brought a soccer ball for young Florencio, and hair combs and lotions from Maria Antonia for Amanda. On this visit, after Amanda wrote her letter saying she wanted to die, her father did not have the look of a man bearing gifts. When they arrived at the house, Florencio, Sr. greeted the other children, then went to check on the livestock. Amanda followed him everywhere he walked.

"Do you know what you are doing to your mother?" Florencio, Sr. asked as he washed his hands and face at the *pila*.

Amanda gave her father a towel to wipe his face and hands. She was quiet and did not respond to his question. What did he mean?

"She is worried about you, the things you wrote in your letter. Why are you telling her this?" Florencio, Sr. asked.

Amanda's face flushed with shame.

"I'm sorry, Papa, I miss Mama. I want to see her," Amanda said.

"This is not the way to go about it. You should apologize to your mother; tell her these things are not true."

Amanda cried with remorse that she had hurt her mother, and she agreed to write an apology letter. Florencio carried the letter back, but Amanda continued to carry guilt for a long time for writing lies that hurt her mother. Guilt piled on abandonment, pressing down on her resentment for Fredy's harsh treatment, and Amanda fled into Maria Antonia's prayer room early one morning to pray. She put her hands on her face and prayed, like her mother always did. She missed her mother and needed the presence of the room to embrace her like Maria Antonia did the night Amanda fell ill with worms that blocked her breathing. Once again, she was short of breath in the prayer room but this time from heaving and sobbing. She wanted to do the right thing, to respect Fredy and obey him, to get right with her mother: but Amanda thought rules were to be tested, bent until sometimes they broke.

Fredy followed rules, kept his word, and enforced what he said. Amanda saw Fredy work very hard in school as a teacher and as a caretaker on the farm. Though Amanda did not know it, Fredy prayed when he was a young boy, deciding to obey God the rest of his life. He taught Amanda the value of learning, helping her develop more integrity and know the value of keeping rules. While she would be hard pressed to admit it, she developed strong character from her experiences with Fredy. He was teaching her to stand up for herself and others.

Deep inside she felt her brother respected the fact that she would stand her ground. She believed what Maria Antonia said, that if you do the right thing God will take care of you. She memorized the Bible text in 1 John 4:18: *"En el amor no hay temor, sino que el perfecto amor echa fuera el temor.* In love there is no fear, for perfect love drives out fear." She repeated over and over again

Joshua 1:9: *"Ya te lo he ordenado: ¡Sé fuerte y valiente! ¡No tengas miedo ni te desanimes! Porque el Señor tu Dios te acompañará dondequiera que vayas.* Have I not commanded you? Be strong and courageous. Do not be afraid; do not be discouraged, for the Lord your God will be with you wherever you go."

She memorized Philippians 4:13: *"Todo lo puedo en Cristo que me fortalece.* I can do all things through Christ who strengthens me." The words seemed to open her heart towards Fredy, so she viewed him differently, if only momentarily. She noticed that when Fredy played soccer, he laughed and smiled. She thought that in his rare moments of apparent happiness, on the soccer field, he was handsome. She thought of him as a good man, because he was a good son to Maria Antonia, and that mattered a lot to Amanda.

Nearly a year went by and Amanda felt a dark cloud was lifting when the school term ended for Christmas break. Florencio, Sr. traveled to La Jigua to help the children pack and make the trip to La Ceiba. When Amanda's father saw her, he said, *"Hola, mi princesa maya.* Hello, my Mayan Princess." Amanda fell into her daddy's arms. His simple words made her feel as if she were forgiven for writing that letter, and she couldn't wait to see Maria Antonia and feel her forgiving embrace as well.

Amanda walked up the hill to *Abuela* Tula's house to say goodbye. For the journey Tula braided Amanda's hair. With her fingers she wove the strands slowly and spoke softly to Amanda: *"Te quiero.* I love you," Tula said.

Florencio, Sr. and the four children boarded the bus bound for La Ceiba, and a few neighbors came out to say goodbye. The journey was long with several stops and three bus changes. When they stopped in Tela, a city on the north coast, Amanda got off the bus at a store where they could go to the restroom. The coast bustled with commerce, people hauling bananas, pineapples, and coconuts in carts to market. The wind from the shore carried a pungent oceanic odor Amanda had never smelled before, and soon she would stand on the beach of the Caribbean Sea for the first time in her life. More than seeing the beach, Amanda longed to see Maria Antonia. But how would Maria Antonia treat her now, after what Amanda had said in her letter?

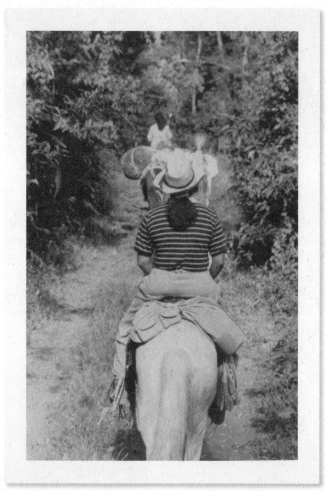

*Dr. Madrid rides into the mountains to treat villagers.*

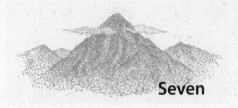

# Seven

# ROMANCING THE STONE

**Doctors—trained to get diagnoses right—are notorious for clashing with other doctors, so a reasonable person might expect two highly-skilled, strong-willed doctors** from different cultures to clash. Drs. Clark and Madrid, however, rarely butted heads. Dr. Madrid had not felt respected and appreciated by many of the men in her life. She enjoyed, however, working with Dr. Clark, who did not condescend but respected her.

Theirs was the rare working relationship where two similar people divided responsibilities and functioned well. In three years the doctors, with the assistance of staff and volunteers, helped Predisan grow from a one-room clinic to three major initiatives: Good Samaritan Clinic, an addiction treatment center, and several small but busy rural clinics.

In 1989 Dr. Clark left Honduras indefinitely to live in the United States. Going through a personal crisis that few fully understood, Robert chose to end his marriage and medical work in Honduras. For months Doris hoped Robert would return to Honduras, but he never came back. With their children in the United States attending university, Doris had to decide whether or not to stay and help run the mission.

Dr. Madrid wondered how the medical mission would continue without Dr. Clark. Would this be the best time for her to pack up and move to La Ceiba? Could she leave without everything caving in? How could a medical organization survive without at least one doctor? Would men respect the leadership of Dr. Madrid without Dr. Clark present?

Even in tearful and bitter months following Dr. Clark's departure, Doris and Amanda knew their biggest challenge was how they would lead Predisan. Similarities between Doris and Amanda ended with the checkbox "female." Perhaps it was Amanda's impulsiveness and carefree nature that distressed Doris, who wanted to know the plan for big projects like the fundraising and building plan for CEREPA. Perhaps Amanda had difficulty accepting the tightly structured environment that Doris believed all the Predisan facilities needed to maintain in order to serve Hondurans well.

In the years following Dr. Clark's departure, however, the two women learned how to balance one another and use their differences to build Predisan. Doris did not allow her loss to prevent her from becoming a strong leader of Predisan. She led relationally and administratively, while Dr. Madrid continued to divide her time between the main clinic, the addiction treatment center, and the rural mountain clinics.

Perhaps the most daunting, Dr. Madrid took up the challenge of traveling as the lone doctor higher into the mountains where no clinics existed.

To help her explore those underserved regions, Dr. Madrid sought the help of a friend named Manny Salazar, the uncle of Diego Salazar. Diego, the one who died defending his village against cartel mercenaries, was a young boy at the time. Manny often took his nephew, Diego, on horseback to the Patuca River to pan for gold. The river contained alluvial deposits of minerals including gold. Manny told Dr. Madrid about the dismal health conditions of the people along the Patuca River.

The news of people suffering and dying for lack of medical care moved Dr. Madrid to recruit staff and volunteers to travel with her to explore the establishment of a medical clinic in the Patuca River region. She enlisted Doña Lola, a Honduran nurse whose steadfast maturity calmed Dr. Madrid in chaotic situations. Tall and light skinned, many people thought Doña Lola was North American.

Dr. Madrid also enlisted a North American nurse named Celia, whom people thought was Honduran. Hondurans knew Celia as generous, often giving away her possessions. Dr. Madrid thought she contributed as much to Predisan's work as Doris and Dr. Clark.

Also joining the expedition were two United States Peace Corps workers. One was named Bill; Predisan partnered with Peace Corps volunteers like Bill, who lived in Las Delicias, helping people build wood-saving stoves and planting trees. For a North American, Bill's Spanish was impeccable. He lived in CEDECO, the Predisan medical clinic network headquarters in the mountains, where Dr. Madrid gave him a room to stay. The second Peace Corps worker, Sam, was loud and opinionated and did not communicate well in Spanish.

Two Honduran agricultural workers also went with the group to consult with villagers about farming problems in the region.

The group traveled in vehicles high into the mountains until roads turned into horse trails in the region where Predisan established clinics. The team paid locals for use of their horses to travel the next stage of the journey. Nurse Celia owned a few horses and spoiled them like grandchildren, but it would require a dozen horses for the whole expedition. The group mounted horses in the Cuyamel River Valley where Celia lived and trained community health care workers. They rode horses east toward the Patuca River, the longest river in Honduras.

After a day traveling by car and horseback, the group camped and prepared for the next leg of the journey, by river. Manny Salazar kept the horses, while Dr. Madrid paid local men to take the group to their final destination by a boat on the Patuca River. From their twenty-foot canoe, the group could see rainbow-feathered macaws in the canopy of trees above the snaking river as they traveled toward the Caribbean Sea. Some of the group prayed they would *not* see the bushmaster pit viper or other tropical venomous snakes along the way.

The acting guide on the boat was a man named Bernardo Garcia, who brought his teenage son to work an oar or use a machete when needed. They also brought guns, for reasons all men everywhere bring guns on such expeditions, but mostly they brought guns because the region was known for violent, lawless bands of gold dredgers.

Dr. Madrid had met Bernardo when he delivered sick people from the Patuca River to a Predisan clinic. Smart and well-spoken, he became the de facto leader for his village because he cared about sick people and pleaded with Dr. Madrid for a clinic to be established on the Patuca River where he lived.

They traveled on the river half a day to reach the village where they would stay the night. As they approached the shore, they saw an encampment of people sheltered under thin tarp shelters.

Smoke from cook fires billowed above the camp of gold prospectors. If the men were dredging, panning, sifting, and finding
gold in the bottom of their shaker boxes, then they would also
viciously protect their turf. For safety, the group's arrival would
need to be explained to the gold dredgers.

After the boat reached the riverbank and the group climbed
out, Bernardo, wearing a gold chain and cowboy hat, explained
to the prospectors that the group had come for another kind of
prospecting: to assess health and other needs along the Patuca
River. He invited them to an open-air meeting the next day. The
Predisan group would camp along the riverbank nearby. Barrel-
chested and heavy, Bernardo sweated as he helped the group
build a tent with tarps.

Those along the riverbank with a fire gave the group coals to
start their own cook fire to prepare food they had brought along.
They balanced pots on three rocks surrounding the fire to heat
beans, tortillas, and coffee in aluminum cookware.

That night as the expedition team bedded down in their
sleeping bags under the tarp shelters, Dr. Madrid heard gold
prospectors talking angrily but could not understand everything
they said. Voices in response sounded stressed and vengeful. *Were
they drinking? Using drugs?* In her assessment of community
health, Dr. Madrid noted that substance abuse often played a
role in human conflicts and health problems, even in the most
remote regions.

The next day only women gathered for the meeting about
health and agriculture. *Why only women?* Dr. Madrid saw a group
of men panning in the distance, and she walked over to them,
asking them to come to the meeting.

"Why not come and discuss how to bring better health to
villages along the river?" Dr. Madrid asked the men. Some men

listened to Dr. Madrid's plea, saying they'd come for the meeting. Others kept panning and did not come.

Returning from her canvassing, Dr. Madrid saw a man in front of his plastic shelter with a coarse black grinding stone. Seeing the grinding stone the length and width of a dining chair seat and very thick, Dr. Madrid's mind drifted to her childhood. She and her sisters pushed a smaller rock across dried corn contained in the slightly scooped out top of the larger stone. With continued crushing, the girls turned dried corn into cornmeal that would finally be made into tortillas.

"Sell me that stone!"

"Make me an offer," the man replied.

"Three thousand lempiras," Dr. Madrid said.

The man did not reply but pressed his lips together, turned down his mouth, nodding disapproval of the offer. The owner of the grinding stone closed off to Dr. Madrid after she had made her offer. Negotiation ended. How much would she have to offer this man for his grinding stone?

Men the doctor had recruited came and joined the women, sitting on rocks, benches, and on the grass.

Though the meeting had begun, Dr. Madrid couldn't get her mind off the grinding stone. She whispered to one of the local men, "Could you go over and talk to that guy with the grinding stone? I made an offer for the stone, and I think the amount was too low—maybe I offended him."

With her attention split between community health and the grinding stone, Dr. Madrid stood up to address the men and women who had gathered.

"I have a friend who told me about the health conditions here. I came with a group of people who care about community health," Dr. Madrid said, then introduced the group members.

"What are the main health and farming problems you face here?" Dr. Madrid asked.

They listed things that people in developed nations take for granted but people in a poor country lack: a basic clinic, education, clean water, sanitation, ways to control swarms of mosquitoes that spread malaria.

For food, they could grow their own beans and corn. And they had clothing. They dressed in an eclectic mix of whatever they could afford to buy and bring back from markets in cities like Catacamas. Men wore t-shirts or button ups, jeans or work pants, and boots—sometimes mud boots—or any kind of shoe they could afford. Women wore t-shirts or a blouse, skirts, sandals, a closed-toe women's dress shoe, or they walked barefoot. Boys wore shorts while girls more often wore dresses. Many children had no shoes to wear.

The villagers told Dr. Madrid they suffered from diarrhea, fevers, intestinal pain, and weakness. Dr. Madrid knew these were the symptoms of larger community health issues. Open defecation led to human and animal fecal matter sticking to the soles of a barefooted person in the village.

The fecal matter carrying hookworm larvae burrowed into the person's feet. Through the skin, hookworms entered the vascular system of the human host, eventually making their way into the lungs. From the lining of the lungs, hookworms crawled up the trachea, where they were swallowed and entered the digestive tract. In the intestines, hookworms stopped migrating and started reproducing.

One female hookworm alone laid thirty thousand larvae daily, and the feces of the human host carried the larvae out to the community again. When the feces came in contact with soil and people walked on it, the cycle repeated and someone else got infected—this time it was a pregnant woman who had an underweight baby and impaired milk production, and both she and the baby were at risk of death.

The World Health Organization estimates 740 million people worldwide, 44 million of them pregnant, suffer attacks of the hookworm. Two-centimeter-long hookworms poison more people in the jungle than the venomous pit viper.

Didn't shoes solve the problem? Worm medicine? Shoes helped and pills could kill the worms for a season. But neither shoes nor pills attacked the root of the problem: feces on the ground. In communities like this one, one thing stopped hookworms in their deadly tracks: pit latrines.

As they continued to discuss health issues in the village, everyone at the meeting was startled when they heard a distant pop, pop, pop.

Locals told Dr. Madrid that they'd recently killed a wild pig and roasted it. Was someone shooting at another wild pig?

Another loud series of pops reverberated, but this time the shots seemed closer. When Dr. Madrid looked around she saw the man she had sent to negotiate about the grinding stone. He had an AK-47, but he ran into the river. *What was going on?* No self-respecting man with an AK-47 runs from a wild pig. That's food.

Was the camp being attacked? Raiders from across the Nicaraguan border had struck here before. Was the camp being stormed to steal gold?

Pop! Pop! Pop! Pop! Pop!

Dr. Madrid wheeled around and saw another man with an AK-47. It was their contact and host, Bernardo!

Good! Their guide would protect them from raiders. She started to run toward Bernardo, to ask him what was happening, when a woman screamed.

The terrified woman staggered toward the doctor at the meeting area. The woman was pregnant. The doctor had seen her earlier that day and learned she was close to delivery.

Dr. Madrid looked at the woman's heaving chest and saw dark red blood coming through her blouse. The pregnant woman had been shot in the chest.

A young boy ran to the woman's side, urging her to sit down. As he helped her to the ground, the boy said, "Don't die, don't die."

The group had medical supplies, so the doctor and Celia attempted to get an IV started in the woman's arm. As Celia held the IV, Dr. Madrid cradled the pregnant woman. Seeing the amount of blood loss, the doctor thought there was little chance she was going to live. As the woman faded and went limp in the doctor's arms, Dr. Madrid felt the woman's bulging abdomen—the baby! She had to get the baby out!

Dr. Madrid had a pocketknife, and she prepared to take the baby by C-section.

Meanwhile, Honduran agricultural workers and Bill the Peace Corp worker were frantically entreating locals to tell them what was going on. The other Peace Corp worker, Sam, ran for cover in the jungle. Doña Lola was in shock, retreating to the flimsy makeshift plastic shelter. Nurse Celia was by Dr. Madrid's side.

A man with a gun came and pointed at Celia, ordering her to help a man who was shot. She looked at the doctor for a directive.

"Go, help him!" Dr. Madrid told Celia, so she went.

Dr. Madrid felt for the pregnant woman's pulse. She had none. Dr. Madrid reached for her knife and unbuttoned the pregnant woman's blouse to begin cutting.

"Don't do it," a man said.

Amanda looked up. The voice was that of the oldest of boat pilots.

"But we need to get this baby out!" Dr. Madrid said, holding the knife inches from the woman's belly.

"Do not do this," the boat pilot said.

"But she's dead! We need to get this baby out, now!"

"No, do not do it. When the husband sees what you've done, he's going to think you killed her," he said.

"The baby!" Dr. Madrid said.

What was Dr. Madrid supposed to do? She knew from talking with the woman earlier in the day that the pregnancy was close to full term. Two cuts and she could have the baby out and breathing. She took an oath to do no harm, to help everyone, and she had to do this. What should she do?

"You're just going to get yourself in big trouble," the boat pilot said.

She held the knife over the woman's belly.

Could the baby survive out here after a traumatic entrance into the world?

Who would care for the baby?

Was it irresponsible to try to do this with non-sterile instruments? Could the baby get infection and die anyway?

Dr. Madrid sighed deeply. She closed the knife and went to help Celia with the second gunshot victim.

Bullets had shredded the man's arm and side, but he was still alive. They had to stop the bleeding. Celia and the doctor wrapped his wounds, but he needed to be transported to a hospital soon.

"I'm going to find Bernardo. He can take him to the hospital down river," Dr. Madrid said, and she ran to find their guide.

When the doctor found Bernardo, he was standing next to a large tree, pointing his AK-47 at a bleeding man on the ground, a third victim.

She approached Bernardo with open palms, her face scrunched in confusion. "What's going on?" Dr. Madrid asked.

"This guy ruined my life," Bernardo said.

"You *shot* him?" she said.

"He wanted to shoot me!" Bernardo replied.

*What!? Was Bernardo—their guide!—the first to attack?*

Dr. Madrid got on her knees to check the second man's pulse. Nothing. He was dead. Bernardo nudged the doctor away.

"Make sure he's dead," Bernardo told his son.

"What?" Amanda said. "He's already dead! Leave him alone!"

"I want to know he's dead!" Bernardo said.

In that moment the doctor understood she'd put herself and her group of medical and agricultural workers at risk in the hands of a loco. Now the expedition was affiliated with a killer in a strange place in the remote mountains.

"Give me your gun. You could injure someone!" Dr. Madrid realized part of what she'd said was ridiculous. He already *had* injured or killed three people.

"What?! I'm not going to give you this gun," Bernardo said. Then Bernardo cut a piece of the man's ear and put it in his pocket.

This added to Dr. Madrid's confusion. *What was going on with Bernardo? Now, who would take the other man to the hospital?*

"Why don't we pray?" Dr. Madrid said, pulling Bernardo's arm.

Strangely, Bernardo agreed. Dr. Madrid returned to Celia, then together they coaxed Doña Lola out from the shelter, telling her the gun battle was over. The doctor called the Peace Corps workers, the agricultural consultants, and the prospectors together.

While Dr. Madrid prayed, Bernardo held his AK-47, looking nervously around the group. Dr. Madrid and a few others prayed with their eyes open to watch for what Bernardo might do.

After the prayer, Bernardo and his son walked briskly toward the riverbank to the group's boat, tied up alongside other wooden motorboats.

"Where are you going?" Dr. Madrid called to Bernardo. No reply. The doctor ran after them.

Catching up to them, panting, she asked, "What are you doing?"

"I'm taking the boat," he said. He moved toward the group's boat.

"You cannot take our boat! First we need to take this injured man to the hospital," she said. "And what about our group? We're here because you invited us; how can you do this and leave us out here?"

"People know who you are, and people are not going to hurt you, but if I stay here another minute someone's going to kill me."

Bernardo aimed his gun at the gas containers in the other boats on the riverbank, but Dr. Madrid interrupted his shot, nearly throwing herself in front of Bernardo's rifle.

"What are you doing?!" Dr. Madrid asked.

"I don't want anybody to follow me," Bernardo said.

"Don't you do that! We can't get out of here if we don't have fuel," Dr. Madrid said.

Doña Lola screamed at Dr. Madrid to get out of the way and let him leave or the doctor was going to get herself—and maybe others—shot.

"Nobody is going to follow me! I'm destroying all the fuel containers," Bernardo said.

Then Bernardo leveled his rifle at the gas cans in other boats, firing a bullet into each container, and the precious fuel for boats to leave this remote region spilled out into the hulls.

Between shots into each of several boats on shore, Dr. Madrid still tried to stop him. "Bernardo, you cannot do that!"

Dr. Madrid said. She called on God to give her something, anything to stop their guide gone berserk. *What do I say, God!?
What do I do!?*

He was still attempting to fire bullets in the remaining
fuel containers when Dr. Madrid said, "I have three gringos
here from the United States. If anything happens to them, the
United States Marines are going to search the jungle to find
you. I hate to think what they would do to you and your son!"
Dr. Madrid screamed at Bernardo.

Bernardo had his gun leveled, ready to finish off the final
gas cans, but he lowered his rife. "Really?" he said.

"This has to do with North Americans now, and you don't
want to mess with them."

"Maybe you're right," Bernardo said, "but promise me you
won't let anyone chase me."

"I promise."

The doctor, however, did *not* let Bernardo take the group's
boat. He and his son escaped on foot, hacking their way through
the jungle, close to the riverbank to the next village. Dr. Madrid
learned later that Bernardo and his son had reached the next
village, pointed a gun at a boat owner's head, and comman-
deered a boat to escape.

They sent the man with the side wound by another boat to
the Moravian Hospital on the Mosquito Coast about fifty miles
away. With a second boat villagers returned the body of the
pregnant woman who had been shot in the chest to her home
area a few miles away. As they loaded the woman's lifeless body
with the baby still inside, Dr. Madrid watched, wiping tears
from her eyes.

Only the body of the man Bernardo killed remained. What
would they do? The other two boat pilots said they were related
to the man, that they were duty-bound to take the body.

"We're taking the boat," the oldest man—the one who'd told Dr. Madrid not to open up the pregnant woman—said. "We can't take your group back in the boat."

"Yes, you *are* taking us back!" Dr. Madrid said.

"We're family to the man who was killed. We want to return his body to his wife and parents for burial," the old man told Dr. Madrid.

"Okay, but how long will it take you to transport this body?" Dr. Madrid asked.

The men told the doctor it could be hours, or maybe the next day before they returned. Dr. Madrid thought for a moment, then said, "Take the body, but you *will* come back to get us, and you *will not* chase Bernardo!"

As insurance, she said one of pilots must stay. She also sent one of the group's agricultural workers with the boat. She wanted to make doubly sure this boat pilot came back for them, and quickly.

The older boat pilot agreed he would not chase Bernardo. The other pilot agreed to stay. The two men made a piece of twine from a plant fiber, tied the twine to the dead man's feet, wrapped him in a blanket, then they carried the body to the boat.

What the group witnessed—the tying of a twine to the man's feet—was a sign that the killer would not get away with this. It was a curse on the killer. But Bernardo had already cut a piece of the dead man's ear off, an effort to counteract the inevitable curse. The belief was that the killer would eat the piece of his victim's ear in order to make the counteraction take effect.

After the boat pilot and the doctor's trusted ally departed with the corpse, the group was left in the upper mountain jungles with no form of transportation. No one—locals or the group—felt they could hold any further meetings. Traumatized, they could no longer imagine coming back here and holding clinics—not in this place, not this particular group of medical and agricultural staff.

A group state of shock settled over them like a late afternoon fog ringing a mountain peak. Dr. Madrid knew she had to lead, to figure out what they would all eat, where they would sleep and feel safe. She had to focus. They prayed and sang spiritual songs to help calm everyone. She dismissed the group to gather their belongings to leave later that day or in the morning.

The doctor sighed deeply. She did not pack her own things yet. Instead, a mysterious preoccupation returned to her. She still wanted the grinding stone. She found the tent of the owner, and a young boy about ten years old was inside.

"Will you sell me the stone?" Dr. Madrid asked the boy.

Celia and Doña Lola walked to the banks of the river in front of the tent where Amanda was talking to the boy. From a short distance, they motioned her over, interrupting the negotiation for the stone.

"What are you doing?" Doña Lola asked.

"I want that stone. It reminds me of—"

Doña Lola stopped her. "Don't you care about us being killed here? Just forget about that stupid stone and help us get out of here!" Doña Lola said.

"We'll get out of here, just calm down," Dr. Madrid told the nurse, and she returned to her negotiation with the boy.

"What's your price?" she asked.

The boy gave her a price that she could live with, and it was a deal. She hoped she had enough money and wouldn't have to ask the nurses, particularly now that they'd objected to her romancing the stone. From her pockets and saddlebags, she had enough to pay the boy. But when the doctor tried to pick up the stone, she had to call for help. And she realized they would have to pack the fifty-pound mammoth out of the jungle by boat and horseback!

Meanwhile, the group learned of a Honduran government headquarters house nearby where they monitored the level of the river for a hydroelectric power project downstream. Dr. Madrid sent Peace Corp workers, Bill and Sam, up the hill, and they quickly spotted the government house. It would provide a safe house for the group.

One of the mountain residents helping the group panicked, saying the relatives of those who were killed would come and take revenge against them because they were Bernardo's friends.

"After the shootings, I saw you hugging Bernardo! They'll think we are his friends and come for us!" the man said.

"I wasn't hugging him! When I realized he was killing, I tried to prevent him from killing others. I was trying to calm him down—that's why I put my hands on him!" Dr. Madrid told the frightened man.

The group was still on edge when they reached the government house. They dropped their packs on the grassy grounds around the house. The caretaker was informed of their plight, and he allowed them to shelter for the night under the porticos of the house. They prayed and read from the Psalms as the sun set on the tragic day.

Seeing that Doña Lola was still in shock, Dr. Madrid put her in charge of cooking for the group, believing the activity and responsibility would settle her nerves.

The caretaker had a two-way radio, and Dr. Madrid suggested that the other agricultural worker in the group transmit a distress signal to the Mosquito Coast.

"Just say that we are in Tropical Lanza and need help, then repeat it," Dr. Madrid said.

The agricultural worker delivered the message, raising the pitch and urgency in his voice with each repetition: "Tropical Lanza to Mosquito Coast? We have an emergency!" Nothing.

"Tropical Lanza to Mosquito Coast, come in Mosquito Coast, over!"

No response.

After repeating the distress call for an hour with no response, Dr. Madrid said, "Why don't you just say, 'We're on Patuca River and we have found a mine of gold and we will share with whoever helps us get out of the jungle.'" He looked at Dr. Madrid, puzzled, thinking she was serious, then finally laughed.

As night fell, each person agreed to take a turn staying awake to guard the group. Dr. Madrid was exhausted but she couldn't sleep. She reclined in a hammock most of the night, hearing the gunshots in her head over and over, remembering what it felt like having a pregnant woman die in her arms, questioning her decision not to cut her open to save the baby.

Guilt pierced her like the gunshot in the pregnant woman's chest. The harrowing experience would eventually cause the doctor to have recurring nightmares about the unseen baby. Each time she had the dream, she woke with the lingering, sick feeling that she could have or should have saved that baby. Had she done the right thing? Should she have allowed the man's comment about getting in trouble with the woman's husband to enter her decision?

When dawn finally broke, roosters crowed and macaw parrots belted out "ack, ack!" in the thick tree canopy above them. Few of the group members felt like eating or drinking, but Dr. Madrid insisted—they would need their strength for the return trip. Besides, they had time. The boat had not arrived. They should eat.

From their provisions, Doña Lola and Celia warmed tortillas on a small pan and smeared them with reddish bean paste.
They heated water for coffee, and the warm drink in the cool
of the morning soothed the group members.

Finally the two men returned. The group loaded the boat
then set off from the riverbank. Just as they were shoving off,
the former owner of the grinding stone and the boy ran to the
group's boat. They were pointing and waving for them to wait,
to come back to shore.

"See, Amanda! He wants his stone back!" Doña Lola said.

They didn't want the stone but they did want a ride. The boat
pilot slowed the motor.

"We're sorry," the boat pilot told the man and the boy, "we
can't take strangers; too much has happened—we don't know
who might be chasing you."

Before the motor revved and they continued on, Dr. Madrid
heard the man saying to the boy, "I told you not to sell her that
stone! We could have exchanged it for a ride in the boat!" Instead,
the stone rode between Dr. Madrid's feet on the floor of the boat.

Dr. Madrid rubbed her hand across the rough and pitted
surface of the ancient lava stone. The grinding stone reminded
her of the one at her grandmother Tula's house, how as a girl she
took her turn crushing corn into fine powder. Now, she felt like
corn on the grinding stone. In the words of 2 Corinthians 4:8-10,
she felt "hard pressed on every side, but not crushed; perplexed,
but not in despair; persecuted, but not abandoned; struck down,
but not destroyed."

Dr. Madrid thought about trying to find Bernardo, to try
and understand exactly what happened. She never saw Bernardo
again, but his angry red face burned in her memory. Still, she had
no clue how she would report on all this—to her supporters, to
the police, to her family members.

She had watched Bernardo hovering over a dying man who had "ruined his life." *How did all that killing un-ruin Bernardo's life?*

As the boat traveled upriver, returning to the horses, the vehicle, then home to Catacamas, one scene played over and over in the doctor's mind. Before Bernardo and his son disappeared into the jungle, they had returned to the bleeding man by the tree. Dr. Madrid had heard Bernardo tell his son, "Kill him!" He did not waste another bullet, like the ones wasted on the gas cans. Instead, he ordered his son to finish the man with a machete. The man was long dead but the teenager did what he was told.

After all that happened, how could the doctor establish a health clinic in such a distant and dangerous place?

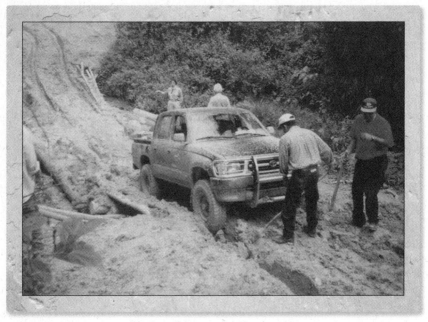

*Truck stuck on mountain jungle roads.*

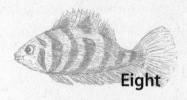

# Eight

# FORBIDDEN

**Amanda traveled by bus with her father and three siblings from the state of Copán east through the industrial center, San Pedro Sula, on a road that passes between the Pico** Bonito Mountains and the shores of the Caribbean Sea to the northern coast fruit-exporting town called La Ceiba.

She felt the embrace of the mountains to the right and beach to the left of her. Amanda felt as if she had fled the land of ruins—Copán—and arrived on the coast of freedom: La Ceiba. The name of the town comes from a mammoth Ceiba tree with exposed roots like fins on the base of a rocket the height of two men; the limbs spread like a mama with saggy triceps, protecting the laborers resting from loading tons of "yellow gold" from trains onto ships in the port.

Honduras was known as a "banana republic" because companies like Standard Fruit de Honduras, started by three Sicilian brothers in 1899, and United Fruit Company, now Dole, controlled the politics and purse strings of the small fledgling nation more than the politicians. The city was bustling in 1966, with tens of thousands of workers planting, cutting stalks, carrying, loading on trains, offloading from train to ship—all gently—because most girls Amanda's age in the United States would not eat the bananas with bruises.

Reuniting with her family in this cosmopolitan city, Amanda saw relief in her father's and mother's eyes. Florencio, Sr. told the children that the house and land in Copán would be sold to his brothers. The family would live in a house in La Ceiba town, but Florencio, Sr. had also bought a farm fifty-five kilometers east of the city in a village called El Cacao. Citrus trees, date palms, and coconut trees already grew on the farm. A wise farmer and a shrewd businessman, Florencio, Sr. grew cash crops that big businesses had still not monopolized for export, as they had bananas and pineapples. He sold milk to local producers, date palms for oil producers, and oranges from his grove of trees to local exporters.

Because of the farm's success and Maria Antonia's concern for the children they'd left behind, Amanda and the other three children who had stayed in the state of Copán would move to La Ceiba permanently. This was the most exciting Christmas of Amanda's life, a permanent reunion with her family.

A few days before Christmas, Florencio, Sr. drove the family in his station wagon to the farm in El Cacao. Maria Antonia hired extra workers for the days of preparation for the Christmas meal. Outside the modest adobe farmhouse, in the shelter for cooking, next to the *pila,* several women helped Maria Antonia slow roast a whole pig over a spit. The next day the women filled a pot belly cauldron full of tamales that they had stuffed with the pork, wrapping each tamale with banana leaves that were plentiful around the farm. In the cauldron over the fire, the tamales steamed and produced an aroma that aroused the appetite of neighbors like the smell of charcoal grilled steaks swirling in a neighborhood.

The hired ladies could manage the cooking while Maria Antonia doted on Amanda and soothed the guilt she felt leaving the four children behind. She presented Amanda with a new yellow flower print dress to wear to church on Christmas Eve.

Smelling, anticipating, and tasting Maria Antonia's tamales, hearing the younger children playing, the older siblings joking, holding her ears for the bang of the firecrackers, wearing a new dress, and sitting at the full table with happiness all around her at the farm, Amanda felt she was home.

After sharing a long meal together on Christmas Eve, the family went to the church Florencio, Sr. had started in El Cacao, and some of the siblings acted in Christmas dramas. The tradition they'd followed in Honduras was to stay up past midnight to welcome in Christmas Day together, saying "Feliz Navidad."

On Christmas day at the farmhouse, the Madrid family sang hymns and Christmas carols as neighbors and family members stopped in throughout the day. Florencio, Sr. hired a dancing troupe to entertain the family and neighbors. The dancers were *Garifuna*—people who trace their roots to West Africa and live along the northern coast of Honduras, the island of Roatán, and other Central American countries. The women moved their hips in a circular motion in a dance of celebration called the *punta* while men played a large bass and a smaller tenor drum.

Uncharacteristic of Florencio, Sr. he danced with the troupe, and everyone laughed. Seeing her father dance, Amanda knew he was happy. The family had endured a difficult year and held together.

As Amanda entered high school, her parents decided she and the other children would have the best possible education, which meant attending the Catholic school in La Ceiba. Maria

Antonia was happy with Amanda attending Catholic school. Florencio, however, suspected a Catholic conspiracy to keep people in ignorance rather than teaching them to read and study the Bible for themselves.

On school nights in their home in La Ceiba, Florencio, Sr. sat down with Amanda while she studied at the kitchen table. Amanda knew her father's misgivings about Catholics, but Amanda had many Catholic friends.

"What are Catholics doing that's so wrong?" Amanda asked her father.

"They have mass in Latin and do not teach people to read the Bible. They have many icons but they become like idols," Florencio said. "In the Ten Commandments, the Lord said, 'Thou shalt not make unto thee any graven image!'"

"I'll pay you to read the Bible," Florencio told Amanda.

Amanda agreed, and Florencio regularly tested her knowledge, book by book, chapter by chapter, before paying her small amounts. By age fourteen, Amanda had read the whole Bible. These table talks strengthened the bond with her father, though she'd argue with him on points of doctrine taught by Evangelical churches, like the one Florencio, Sr. led as a lay pastor.

At Amanda's school, San Isidro, a short bus or bike ride down palm tree lined streets from the Madrid home in La Ceiba, she could feel the breeze from the Caribbean and see beaches and ports.

One day Amanda's religion and music teacher, a young monk in his twenties, took his class to the beach where he played his guitar while the teenagers sang along. He relied on Amanda for a repertoire of "evangelical" songs that he allowed her to teach the other students.

Florencio, Sr. talked to the headmaster about Amanda not attending daily mass because of the family's Pentecostal beliefs, and the priest allowed this because he wanted to administer mass only to Catholics, not the unwilling or non-Catholics. This was the Madrid family's way of standing firm in their beliefs; this kind of staunchness extended into the classroom, where Amanda enjoyed debate with her fellow students, even the teachers. Her philosophy teacher, an attorney, quoted ancient Greek philosophers or church fathers, applying the teachings to Honduran life and experience. They studied great theologians and thinkers like Blaise Pascal and Augustine, and she latched on to Pascal's idea that the heart has reason that reason cannot know and Augustine's notion that the human heart is restless till it finds rest in God.

From that very first day of schooling in La Jigua as a very young girl where she told God she would give her life to him, Amanda had been restless to know more about her creator. So Amanda enjoyed philosophy most because the teacher would not simply lecture but engage in discussion. Often he would say, "Let's hear what Amanda thinks."

She became a leader among her peers, writing and debating about gender issues. In her teen years she began in earnest what she had experienced earlier in the tension with her brother—her quest to understand what she could do as a woman. If she didn't have equal physical strength to a man, what did she have? A woman cannot build like a man, but a man cannot build love in the heart of a child like a woman. She imagined she would someday be married and have many children like Maria Antonia. But she also wanted to fulfill a deep desire to help others, and the way she envisioned that happening was by being a doctor who healed people. She could be respected because, at the worst of times for a human being, the doctor is there to bring life back to equilibrium.

While she was exempt from attending the daily mass, Amanda loved the icons and architecture of the Catholic Cathedral for the same reasons she loved the *Viernes Santo y la Procesión y Fiesta* (Good Friday Procession and Fiesta) that she attended against her father's wishes many years ago in La Jigua. Every day the Catholics rang a bell to call students and townspeople to mass. They had statues and icons, and the cathedral was more airy and light than the small Evangelical churches in which she'd sat for long hours. And the Catholics had wine.

The cathedral was always open, so parishioners and students were encouraged to enter, to pray anytime they felt the need. One day Amanda's classmates went in, ostensibly to pray. Instead, they explored and discovered the unlocked storage room for the communion wine.

They found a glass and poured small shots to drink the altar wine, as if it were a toast to being liberated. After drinking, they filled the bottle back to the full line with water from the tap nearby.

The Catholic priests would consider anathema the girls stealing the holy wine, drinking without the sacramental observances and the priest administering it. Amanda's Evangelical friends thought drinking wine in a Catholic church in any case would be abhorrent. Amanda had sinned by standards of Catholics and Evangelicals.

Very soon after the girls had their fun with sips of wine and refilling with water, all the students at San Isidro Catholic High School received a homily about the evils of tampering with the altar wine and a warning that the perpetrators, when caught, would be expelled from school. The girls were never caught, never expelled, but the cost of those few giggling moments with her friends was the wincing memory of drinking the forbidden fruit. Quietly a thorny vine grew and wrapped around Amanda's conscience.

Amanda was not as religious as her family may have wanted. She didn't mind going to church, but she hated the nonsense rules.

As long as the preachers told good stories from the Bible and stayed away from their harangues against her Catholic friends, she was mildly agreeable to the multiple meetings in the church each week.

Florencio, Sr. read the Bible aloud to all the children in the Madrid home, selecting a psalm for the day or reading a story from the Gospels or the Old Testament. Maria Antonia and Florencio, Sr. would alternate leading the devotionals, so Amanda often heard her mother's soothing reading voice as well as her father's. Maria Antonia quickly developed a reputation—as she did in Copán—as a leader known for her ministry of praying for the sick. In Amanda's eyes, Florencio, Sr. did more teaching and Maria Antonia did more to live the teachings of Jesus.

Florencio, Sr. and Maria Antonia also taught the children to pray, and they'd call on them to pray for their siblings. If Amanda had an unresolved argument with a sibling, she'd leave out the name of that brother or sister when she prayed.

"Dad! Did you hear that? Amanda did not pray for me!" the sibling would complain.

In the evenings, on certain nights of the week in La Ceiba, the family would gather and listen to a radio program called "The Unchained Life." It told stories of people whose bondage to sin was broken by God, and they were freed from the snare of money, addiction to drugs, or alcohol. They said religion was the answer, but Amanda had plenty of that, more than she thought she needed, really.

Amanda wanted to be free, too. Those stories she heard on the radio shaped Amanda's young faith and future choices. She remembered them more than the sermons of local preachers, though she enjoyed hearing from one young traveling preacher whose name was Don Coronado.

Don Coronado rode into town on a mule, and when he dismounted he stood barely taller than Amanda. Like Amanda's grandfather, Gregorio, Don Coronado was a short man with Mayan features and light skin. He wore a bowler hat, rounded and not angular like the cowboy hats Honduran men wore. He had a small moustache, and Amanda thought he was cute. She was attracted to him not so much for his handsomeness as for his alluring mix of spirituality and rugged simplicity. She was curious about Don Coronado, a mystic of sorts who seemed to supersede religious sectarianism and radiated godliness freely like the salty sweat that soaked his bowler hat. She admired how he'd never take leave of anyone without asking, "Do you have a prayer request?"

When Amanda was very young, Don Coronado prayed for Amanda, placing his hands on her head and lifting his voice up to God. The prayer renewed a fire in her soul to please God who heard her cry for help in the outhouse the first day of school in Copán. When Don Coronado prayed for Amanda, she felt a sense of security. Amanda had some money she'd made selling seeds to the local grocer, so she donated to Don Coronado, feeling she was paying her dues for the holy man's prayers.

She felt good to help support his preaching. She now understood why so many people liked to host Don Coronado in their homes while he stayed in their town. He would stay in the Madrid home and talk late into the night with Florencio about Bible topics, and Amanda would listen until she could not stay awake any longer. After a few days in the Madrid home, the itinerant preacher mounted his mule and rode to the next town.

Don Coronado represented the mystical free spirit Amanda wanted to be. The Pentecostal Church, on the other hand, was too restrictive for Amanda. Her free spirit was stifled there. She resented her family's church because she was forbidden to wear pants, forbidden to accept if she was ever elected "Queen of the Barrio," forbidden to have a *quinceañera* like the Catholics girls did at age fifteen, forbidden to participate in dramas having to do with holy days and Catholicism. For Amanda, her church experience could be summed up in one word: *Prohibido!* Forbidden!

Compounding her resentment, Amanda felt she had to be perfect in church, because Florencio, Sr. was a lay pastor. She couldn't wear makeup or earrings, because those things were sinful adornments unbecoming of a young girl. Pants were also questionable for girls, and Amanda had a pair of green pants she really liked.

"You may not wear those pants in church," Florencio said.

"What's wrong with wearing pants in church?" Amanda asked.

"It's wrong."

"What's wrong with wearing pants? Where does the Bible say that?"

He read from Deuteronomy 22:5: "The woman shall not wear that which pertaineth unto a man, neither shall a man put on a woman's garment: for all that do so are abomination unto the LORD thy God."

"Now," Florencio, Sr. continued, "do you think you will wear those pants to church?"

The verse confused Amanda. How could bright green pants "pertaineth unto a man"? No man would want to wear these green pants. Amanda stayed quiet, pausing the argument for the moment. But secretly she had a plan.

The day of the next church gathering, Amanda put on her green pants, and after her father was already standing in front of the congregation to preach, she walked down the center aisle to the front row and sat down. Her bright green pants seemed to glow. She pursed her lips, squinted her eyes slightly, crossed her legs, and looked at her father.

Florencio, Sr. did not point out his daughter. He did not stop in mid-sentence. He did not send Amanda out of church and back home to change. He continued to teach, and Amanda sat wondering what he thought. But he never satisfied her with a response to her open challenge. He did not talk about it for months, until Amanda finally asked and her father said he'd rather have his daughter in church wearing bright green pants than outside the church in a dress.

During her high school years Amanda searched on the ragged edges of orthodox Christianity, looking beyond her mother's Catholicism and her father's Pentecostalism. She attended gatherings or studied beliefs of Mormons, Jehovah's Witnesses, 'Baha'i, Ancient and Mystical Order of Rosae Crucis, and Ecclesia Gnostica.

Florencio, Sr., meanwhile, not only wanted Amanda in the church but wanted her to stay in La Ceiba after she graduated and to work for her brother, Fredy, as his secretary. Amanda's father even enrolled her in secretary's school, which she attended during her last terms of high school. She did not want to be a secretary, much less Fredy's secretary.

One day Amanda and her father were sitting together at the kitchen table.

"Papa, I want to go to university and medical school," she said.

In Honduras medical school is more integrated into the university years of study, rather than a separate school after a four-year university degree. The first year of university studies in the medical program, however, is for general studies, and the second year is more focused on chemistry and biology.

"You can go to university in La Ceiba," Florencio told Amanda. This would allow her to work for Fredy while also working on her university degree.

"I was thinking of university in Tegus," Amanda said.

Florencio was protective of his Mayan Princess. He could not imagine his daughter going off to the big city of Tegucigalpa for university, but he did not explain how he feared for her life, her morality, her soul in a big city. Instead, he simply forbade her to go.

"No, I will not support you to go to Tegus," Florencio said. His decision was final. Amanda knew she had to get her plans on the table. She was deeply hurt by not receiving her father's blessing, but she knew it might come to this kind of impasse, so she had been saving money for living expenses and university fees in Tegucigalpa.

"I already have my plan and I do not need your support," Amanda told her father.

She had declined getting luxuries such as a class graduation ring or dresses for celebrations, instead saving money for university and medical school fees. She worked as a salesperson in a store, making good sales commissions. In many Latin American families it might be expected that she share her earnings, but she was allowed to open a bank account and save the money for her own use. She went to their farm and brought back coconuts, eggs, citrus fruits, and corozo nuts that buttons are often carved from, and she sold them in the market in La Ceiba. She was grateful to her father for allowing her to save money, even though he did not know how she planned to use it. As *Abuela* Tula often said, "*Viva para el pisto*. They are good to make money."

The day Amanda turned eighteen, she got her identity card, her driver's license, and an independent bank account at Atlántida, the oldest bank in Honduras, and she transferred the money she'd saved in a parent-child account into the independent one.

Florencio, Sr. had been at the farm for weeks for harvesting, and he returned to La Ceiba to see Amanda on her birthday. On his arrival Amanda informed her father, "I'm leaving next week for medical school in Tegus." She found it difficult to look her father directly in the eyes because this news would be like telling him she was going to die next week. When she cut her eyes at him, she saw fear and a twinge of anger. He left Amanda and hastily searched for Maria Antonia.

"She's crazy," Florencio told Maria Antonia. "*Loca*."

All Amanda could think, meanwhile, was that her father didn't trust her, didn't think she was capable of medical school. She ignored or couldn't fathom Florencio's concerns for his precious daughter. Maria Antonia asked Amanda to come into her bedroom. They sat on Maria Antonia's and Florencio's bed.

Maria Antonia did not waste words.

"*Dime*. Tell me."

"I have saved money," Amanda said, beginning to list the reasons she should go to medical school in Tegucigalpa.

Maria Antonia nodded and let her continue.

"I have a bank account. I've been accepted to university in Tegus. I will see Jesús there and he can protect me," Amanda said, referring to her older brother. She lifted her chin slightly, waiting for her mother's reply.

Maria Antonia took a deep breath, sighed, and looked at Amanda. Maria Antonia wiped her nose with a handkerchief.

"*Mi Muñeca*, it sounds like you have a good plan," Maria Antonia said.

Amanda nodded. She believed her plan was foolproof.

"Promise me two things, Amanda. One, you will behave according to the values we have taught you. Two, that if something happens, you will call me."

Amanda felt her mother's trust and blessing like a soothing ointment on burned skin. This trust, for the moment, bridged the canyon of her father's disapproval.

The next week Amanda intended to go to the bank to withdraw her money, but she could not find her bank account passbook. Getting a replacement bankbook would take many days, and waiting would cause her to miss registration for medical school. How would she register now? Would she have to wait another year?

That same week, at a going away party for students of her high school, everyone spoke of their university plans, and Amanda was publicly congratulated for heading off to university and medical school. But secretly she was dying inside. Only her close high school friend knew about her dilemma, and after the party her friend took Amanda home to see his father, a humble businessman named Raul Guerrero. Raul, his son, and Amanda sat at a table on the veranda to talk.

"When you get out of medical school," Raul said, "I want you to be my doctor."

*Oh, no. How could she tell him?* Amanda flushed with embarrassment. She dreaded telling any of the adults in her life—her father, who she had brashly told her plans, Fredy who might gloat over the setback because she could be his secretary at least for a year, Maria Antonia who had helped her father agree to the plans!

Raul began telling Amanda about the big city, to be careful on the bus, in the city, what and who to watch out for.

Why was he saying all this? Why did her friend bring her back for this? If he only knew she was not going! She felt like her heart would burst from holding in her emotions.

Then Raul put an envelope on the table and pushed it across to Amanda. What was this? What was he giving her? He nodded and gestured, encouraging her to open the envelope and look inside.

Amanda tore open the envelope, looked inside, and Raul had given her enough money for a bus ticket plus one month of living expenses in Tegucigalpa.

What was this?! How could she take money from him? Even her own father would not give her money! How could this be? Through her tears she protested, said it wasn't right, and how could she take this money? Raul said the money was a loan and that she could either repay it or become his doctor someday. She got up to hug her benefactor and committed to paying the loan back within a month.

Amanda turned to her friend and thanked him. She knew he'd discretely told his father about her dilemma. She sat back down and cried tears of joy that God had provided through this kind man.

Raul had three sons and no daughters. He said if he had a daughter, he'd want her to be just like Amanda. She committed to God and to Raul that she would make good on the kindness of both.

She did not tell her family about the arrangement, but she went to the bus office and purchased a ticket with the money, closely guarding the rest for living expenses and registration fees. Meanwhile, she applied for another bank passbook and would return for it soon.

A few days later, family and friends accompanied Amanda to the bus station in La Ceiba to say goodbye, and she boarded the bus for Tegucigalpa. Buses always reminded her of the day her family left her as a little girl. She felt incapable of pleasing her father and oldest brother, but she would not be denied to act on her plan.

As the bus left the station, Amanda saw Toñita, now nine years old, crying and waving goodbye.

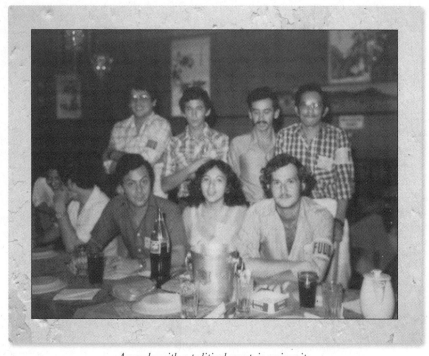

*Amanda with a political group in university.*

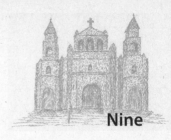

## Nine

# INCREASING PRESSURE

In 1977, Amanda rode the bus into adulthood, an eigh-teen-year-old Mayan farm girl moving to the capital city, her resolve like an arrow. Her dead-straight tenacity would be tested in a city of one million people.

The daylong bus ride from La Ceiba to Tegucigalpa followed switchback roads through folds in soft, rounded mountains, green with trees and terraced crops. The bus traveled over the often steep and winding two-lane highway, meeting logging trucks that thundered like locomotives past teenage boys riding bicycles and balancing bundles of firewood on their handlebars. Pickup trucks sagging with the weight of "just one more" person shared the road with the public bus Amanda was riding in, with laborers on horse or mule-back, with taxis decorated in hand-scribed back windshield sayings like, *Jesus Es Mi Amigo.*

The pressure increased in Amanda's ears as the elevation rose from sea level in La Ceiba to Tegucigalpa's one kilometer. She was anxious to see La Universidad Nacional Autónoma de

Honduras, to see where she would register, get settled, and live. She wondered how she would get along in the big city. She was afraid, but she took comfort in the fact that her brother, Jesús, lived in Tegucigalpa and she would see him soon.

Voices rang in her head, Raul's advice, the cautions from Maria Antonia, and the silence of her father whose fear she sensed about her move to the big city. Pressure was increasing.

Amanda arrived on a Saturday afternoon not knowing where she was going to sleep that night. When she got off the bus, she had directions for a taxi driver to take her to her brother and his friends at a gathering place for Christian young people called Alpha and Omega. The taxi driver hoisted all Amanda owned into the trunk of his small car, then sped through crowded streets, dodging people crossing the street with huge loads heading to the market, weaving around other cars, trucks, buses, and finally pulled up in front of the Alpha and Omega offices. Amanda took a deep breath, paid the driver his fare, and got out of the taxi.

That Saturday afternoon the place was active with people her age gathering for recreation, talking, and Bible study. A few of the leaders knew Amanda as one of the Alpha and Omega leaders from La Ceiba, and they met her at the gate with smiles and open arms.

When she saw her brother, Jesús, she sighed as she fell into his arms. She believed God had already answered her prayers for a new life in Tegucigalpa. Jesús introduced Amanda to other young women. She met Bertha, who insisted Amanda stay at her house, because she too was a new medical school student.

After staying a while at the Alpha and Omega facility, Bertha helped Amanda carry her luggage to the local bus stop down the street. They went to Bertha's house, and Amanda met Bertha's mother, who gave Amanda a bed to sleep on until she could find a permanent place of her own.

Two days later, Bertha and Amanda registered for university. Amanda searched bulletin boards for a place to rent. Weeks passed, then Bertha's mother offered Amanda room and board if she would pay a small rent, cook, and clean. Amanda agreed and stayed.

Eight years of university and medical school training were ahead of her. Each year academic pressure and intensity increased, but in the first few years she had time to join political action groups and a church. She campaigned for her political party's candidates in elections. Her church was largely apolitical. Her medical school, politics, and church were strangely separate and her affections and passions splintered.

In the third year of university, Amanda moved into an apartment with her sister Elsita, who had come to Tegucigalpa for work and to help Amanda through medical school. Beginning the fourth year of university, Amanda took purely medical school courses, just like the ones offered in medical schools worldwide, including the course to weed out the faint of heart and weak of stomach: gross anatomy.

On Valentine's Day 1977, Amanda and her group of medical students received their cadaver for the semester of dissecting and learning the intricate parts of the human body. The group appropriately named their cadaver Valentin, since he came to them on Valentine's Day.

The tall black male was in a long, deep container of formaldehyde, and Amanda dreaded the chore of getting the body in and out of the container each day. She enjoyed the class but the exams were anxiety inducing. The professor would write a question on a card placed on the concrete tables where the cadavers were lying. Sometimes a question was pinned to the body, and Amanda had one or two minutes to identify the part or answer some question related to it. When the teacher rang the bell, students rotated to a different cadaver. Amanda faced difficult tests of character. She endured sexual harassment from the mostly male classmates, and one day a classmate cut the male member off of their cadaver and snuck the body part into Amanda's purse. The sheepishly evil look on a classmate's face the next day told her exactly who had done the shameful act, and though she thought his action asinine, she chose not to report him to the professor.

Amanda saw her first death as a physician while doing clinical rotations. When she witnessed the patient expel his last breath, Amanda cried and left the room, and the attending physician, who was from Spain, followed her into the corridor and scolded her for losing composure.

The same Spanish physician rejected Amanda's examination of a pregnant woman because Amanda said she heard two heartbeats and thought the woman was carrying twins. The use of ultrasound was not yet widespread—Amanda had simply listened with a stethoscope, detecting two fetal heartbeats. Excited, she called for the attending doctor to examine the patient to confirm her opinion, but after listening, he said he only heard one heartbeat. No twins.

The incident deflated Amanda, but medical school thickened her skin. Still, the mistake bothered her. How could she have heard two heartbeats and the attending only one? Was she hearing things? Hours later, after the woman delivered her baby, Dr. Madrid waited for the placenta to emerge, but she saw something else moving inside—another baby! The mother delivered a second baby, and Amanda celebrated for the mother but also felt proud of herself. She rushed to tell the attending doctor the news. Proudly she told him about the twins, implying that he was wrong and she was right. He congratulated her.

Amanda practiced in government and military hospitals in Tegucigalpa with strong academic supervision. Military medicine caught her attention. Without a robust insurance system from which to bill patients, physicians in private practices or hospitals were not always prosperous in Honduras, so the military presented a financially lucrative option for Amanda. In the 1980s, the United States supported the Honduran military and any Central American military movement that opposed or resisted Soviet-supported governments. The military seemed unusually fortified with opportunities during Amanda's time of decision about her future medical career.

Most medical officer positions, however, went to relatives of doctors or high-ranking officers in the army. She wanted a position as medical officer, but she had no relatives in those positions. Not easily deterred, Amanda asked a friend for advice.

"How would a person go about getting a medical assistant position?"

"You need a reference from someone within the military," Amanda's friend, director of military public relations, said. "Do you have a friend or family member in the government?"

"I don't know; is there someone we both know, maybe from our old political party?" Amanda asked.

"Yes, the president of the University of Honduras," the director said, reminding her that the president had mentored their university political group years before.

So Amanda went to the president's office, persisted several days, and she was granted the recommendation. After mountains of personnel paperwork, the Honduran military hired Amanda to be a medical officer.

She earned more money and enjoyed more prestige than ever before. A decade before and against the wishes of her father and brother, Amanda had traveled alone to Tegucigalpa, entered university on a path to medical school, graduated, and now served as one of the few Honduran female doctors. Few women succeeded in the Honduran military, but Amanda proved herself by coordinating immunization and family planning campaigns.

Over the course of her medical service in the Honduran army, she developed an expansive network of friends in government and non-government organizations. Consequently, the military offered Amanda a scholarship to train further outside of Honduras. The scholarship, however, required her to sign on for additional years of service in the Honduran military. She had to make a decision: take the scholarship and remain in debt as a career army doctor, or reject the offer, missing a career opportunity of a lifetime for job security in the military. But would financial security come with a price of her integrity?

One day a lieutenant nicknamed *El Tigre* Bonilla sent a soldier dressed only in his underwear to Dr. Madrid for treatment. Dr. Madrid had no problem treating the patient, but what disturbed her was El Tigre's lack of concern for the man's dignity. She marched into El Tigre's office.

"Why did you send this man to my office dressed only in his underwear? How would you like to be sent to my office wearing only your underclothes?" Dr. Madrid asked.

She'd acted impulsively, and as she stood in front of El Tigre, she was embarrassed she'd barged into his office. She waited for him to pounce. Now she would surely find out firsthand why they called him El Tigre. To her surprise, El Tigre apologized.

Another time while working in the army hospital, Dr. Madrid prescribed an enlisted soldier a particular medicine. When the enlisted soldier went to get the drug at the military pharmacy, the pharmacist turned him away without it. Days passed and the soldier returned, still very ill. Dr. Madrid thought he was taking the medicine she had prescribed. When he made it clear the medicine had not been dispensed by the pharmacy, the news set off alarms in Dr. Madrid's mind. Perhaps there was a logical explanation for this injustice.

Amanda inquired and was told that only officers were allowed the medicine she had prescribed. The more questions she asked, the more she saw her future in the military full of frustration and confrontation.

During her military tenure she learned to shoot a gun. The trainers were happy to see a woman willing to get her hands on weapons, to defend herself and to be an asset rather than helpless in a combat situation.

Honduras at the time had no clear distinction between police and military. They could make war or catch criminals. Dr. Madrid treated criminals when they were hurt while being captured or detained. She saw bloodied criminals and soldiers in the hospital; if one died she also performed the work of a coroner, preparing bodies for the family to identify and claim them.

With the female military police she served an important function of interacting with young women who were in custody or victims of violence. One day two Colombian women came to the hospital complaining of heart problems, so they were brought to Dr. Madrid. She thought they were beautiful and sophisticated looking, and when she examined them discovered their health seemed to be flawless as well. Intuition led Dr. Madrid to wonder what was behind this visit. Both complained of heart symptoms. Neither showed signs of heart problems.

"Tell me the truth," Dr. Madrid said. "What's going on?"

They hesitated. For a moment Dr. Madrid felt the awkward silence of stepping over the line into their personal lives.

"The military is torturing us for information," one of the Colombian women said.

"Tell me."

The women explained that they had been caught up in a string of operations but were not guilty of the things the police accused them of: drug trafficking, money laundering, and prostitution.

"Give us a shot—something, medicine, anything to make us die peacefully."

"I'm not going to do that," Dr. Madrid said, and she went on to talk to the women about the choices they were making and how they could turn their lives around.

What more could she do for them? The interrogators would never admit to any wrongdoing. She felt helpless but also believed God changed the hearts of people and could change the minds of the men prosecuting the two women. Then Dr. Madrid held their hands and prayed for them. The women left and Dr. Madrid never saw them again.

Amanda, who had come to Tegucigalpa from La Ceiba at age eighteen, was now Dr. Amanda Madrid. She was confident in her abilities to diagnose and treat illnesses. As a young physician in training, her disposition was methodical, syllogistic, and industrial and could be expressed in "if-then" statements of cause and effect.

Then tectonic plates shifted under the doctor's feet. The perfect foundation for the life she was building twisted and a crack appeared in the floor the day her sister, Elsita, found a lump on her neck. Dr. Madrid believed with confidence she could solve the problem of Elsita's cancer. If the swelling was here or there, if it was growing or not, it could be this or that, nothing to worry about.

She had rehearsed these syllogisms, the flowcharts, had examined thousands of patients, and was confident she could do something about most anything she saw.

If there was any doubt, tests could be done. Even if results came back showing something life-threatening, she knew how to treat any illness. A biopsy had been done for Elsita, tissue sent to the lab.

Several days later a doctor in the lab handed Dr. Madrid the report. When she looked at Elsita's lab results, her legs became wobbly; she had to sit down. The test paper read "Lymphatic Hodgkins." A highly aggressive and fatal cancer had already spread in her lymph nodes, continuing throughout her body.

"Do you believe this test could be wrong? Could the test plates have been switched with another patient?" Dr. Madrid asked the other doctor.

"No, doctor, the only difference between this diagnosis and the ones you have seen before in the hospital . . . this one is your sister," he said and walked out.

Elsita, Amanda's second mother, was dying. Alone in the sterile lab where answers were supposed to be certain and complete, the flood dams broke and Amanda wept.

The first thing she knew she had to do was tell her sister the results. She discussed with a few of her siblings how much to tell Elsita. Dr. Madrid felt they ought to tell her everything. Other siblings wondered if it would take away her hope for survival to know how far the cancer had spread.

Ultimately Dr. Madrid believed Elsita deserved to know how aggressive the cancer was and that it was in the fourth and most advanced stage. Knowing the extent of the disease would also help in making the decision to get the most advanced treatment possible. Elsita's oncologist and Dr. Madrid revealed everything to her—the full and devastating truth.

Amanda felt powerless, shocked, in denial that her sister was dying. She told Elsita through tears that she had a very aggressive cancer. They held each other and cried. Amanda felt the weight of her sister's care on her shoulders. But everything she knew to do was not enough. There were no easy fixes now. Elsita's cancer was aggressive and fatal. What could Amanda do for her, not just as a doctor but also as a sister?

Elsita, meanwhile, tried to show no fear or worry, for the sake of the family. Her stress, perhaps her attempt to hold all that in, contributed to her developing facial paralysis. Seeing her sister's stress, Amanda began praying for outside help, because she now realized she could not help her sister alone. She cried out to God, "Save my sister!" She prayed for help from other doctors or hospitals. Praying reminded Dr. Madrid the power of life and death belonged not to her as a doctor, but to God.

With the help of friends in North America, Dr. Madrid secured a reservation at MD Anderson Cancer Center in Houston, Texas. The two sisters flew from Tegucigalpa to Houston, where Elsita received chemotherapy and radiotherapy. Though the treatments were difficult, Amanda stayed by her side for three months in Houston.

As they traveled back to Tegucigalpa, exhausted from hospital stays, chemotherapy, and radiology treatments, Amanda thought about what cancer had done physically to her sister, emaciated and bald headed. More profound than physical changes was what happened in the hearts of patient and caregiver. Elsita was Amanda's rock, sturdy like the warm flat stone on the banks of the Juile River in La Jigua. Now Amanda felt as if she had that rock on her shoulders.

Amanda prayed for a miracle for Elsita, for a full healing of her body from the cancer. At a crossroads, she prayed for God to show the way. She'd been in Tegucigalpa twelve years. Four years in university. Four years in medical school and residency. Four years working as an army medical officer. The army wanted her to train further, achieve higher rank, move up, and they made lucrative offers. Some of her family wondered how she could refuse such an offer from the military. What would she do?

Tears streamed down her face as Amanda felt God calling her to make a decision she knew would be unpopular with nearly everyone she knew. Amanda decided not to take the scholarship that would have opened the door for a military career. Against the wisdom of her medical community and family, she was headed to Catacamas.

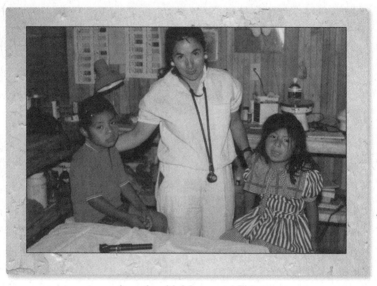

*Amanda with Marcos and Fide.*

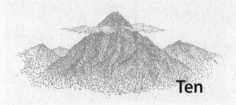

# Ten

# NO PLANS TO DIE

**In early 1989, a woman named Tomasa, dying with cancer, came to Dr. Madrid's house in Catacamas. She looked steadfast, with something on her mind to discuss with** the doctor. Every time she saw Tomasa, Dr. Madrid thought of Elsita's fight with cancer.

Dr. Madrid had been treating Tomasa for months, had sent her to a hospital in Tegucigalpa for consultation with a cancer treatment surgeon. The surgeon concluded Tomasa's cervical cancer was so advanced that surgery was not an option.

After the consult, Tomasa went back to her village, Santa Cruz de Capapan, breaking the news to her family and friends. Responding to the failure of modern medicine to address her problem, Tomasa's husband, Eulalio, hired an alternative healer. He told Dr. Madrid, "I trust you, but if there's any hope for this traditional treatment, we will keep trying it."

The next time Dr. Madrid saw her, Tomasa was thin, struggling to breathe, and dying. In a squalid and unsanitary hut,

Tomasa subsisted on thin soup, herbal concoctions, and water. Dr. Madrid informed the healer that she and the local clinic would take over Tomasa's care.

Dr. Madrid did not want to see Tomasa's family spend money on ineffective treatments for a life-threatening illness like cervical cancer. Neither traditional nor modern medicine could do much to heal Tomasa. The cancer had spread to her bladder and lungs.

Fearing death imminent, Tomasa decided to be baptized, so the church leaders took her to the river to immerse her. Tomasa had peace for her own soul, but she was troubled for her children if the cancer took her life.

Tomasa had come back to Dr. Madrid that day in early 1989 with a burden she believed Dr. Madrid could help her carry.

Dr. Madrid poured coffee and they talked. Tomasa sipped her coffee slowly then broke in to speak. She didn't mince words.

"I'm concerned about my children," Tomasa said.

Dr. Madrid put down her coffee.

"Tell me," Dr. Madrid said.

"I don't want my children to be left in the jungle when I die," Tomasa said.

"I know I'm dying. I know my husband will re-marry, and when he does, I fear for my children. Stepmothers are not good to stepchildren," Tomasa said.

Dr. Madrid nodded agreement. Though Dr. Madrid didn't have children of her own, she felt the pain of leaving four children she loved who were stair step in age: 2, 4, 6, and 8. Dr. Madrid remembered that her own mother, Maria Antonia, had been orphaned. How could she allow four children to face the plight of orphans and stepchildren who often suffer mistreatment?

"I've been praying and thinking about my children—who will care for them after I die? As I pray, Dr. Madrid, your face keeps coming to my mind," Tomasa said.

Dr. Madrid smiled but inside she panicked. Why was she coming to Tomasa's mind? What was she going to ask?!

"I just came to ask you something very important." Tomasa looked Dr. Madrid in the eyes.

"Would you take care of my children when I die?"

Dr. Madrid's body went slack and she nearly dropped her coffee. No! No! Tomasa is not going to do this to her. She couldn't. How could she lay this on her?

Dr. Madrid felt as if she had just taken on a part of Tomasa's cancer. Her stomach felt sick. Her mind raced. How could she take care of a toddler, a four-year-old, a six-year-old, and an eight-year-old? Any age child for that matter!? How could she work full-time as a doctor running a clinic and addiction center in Catacamas, and a growing network of medical clinics in the mountains—and care for children? Four children!

Dr. Madrid wanted to be a mother, but not like this. What can you say to a mother with cancer asking you to care for her children?

"*Tomasa, Si no se preocupe. Yo lo haré.* You don't need to worry. I will do it. I want you to know that the one who adopts them for good may not be me. I will find families for them, I promise you that," Dr. Madrid told Tomasa.

"If you do that, please keep them all together, *Doctora*, I don't want them to be separated," Tomasa said.

Dr. Madrid assured Tomasa that she would do everything in her power to keep the children together. In Honduran culture, it was uncommon to adopt children who were not your family—and to adopt four was unheard of.

They finished their coffee in silence. Tomasa said goodbye, then returned to her village outside Catacamas. Dr. Madrid fell against the closed door, went upstairs, and sat down on the bed, where she would go to talk to God. She was a little girl again, that abandoned girl in front of her house in the state of Copán, watching her mother, father, and siblings leave her and three siblings to live alone in La Jigua. She had to find Tomasa's children a home so they wouldn't fall apart like the four did in Copán. Dr. Madrid and Fredy continued a tense relationship, Elsita had cancer, and Florencio, Jr. was an alcoholic.

What would Maria Antonia advise her to do? She would call her later to ask.

Tomasa went back to her village and told her children they would be going to live with Dr. Madrid. She told them her house was a place of peace and joy, that they would be happy there: a beautiful home with plenty of food, nice beds, and fun things to do. The next time Dr. Madrid went to the mountains to visit, Tomasa said, "Take the children back with you."

But Dr. Madrid believed that taking the children before Tomasa died would signal to the children—to everyone involved— that her motherhood had ended. Being mother of four was Tomasa's last role in life, and Dr. Madrid did not want to take that away prematurely. The doctor renewed her promise to care for the children no matter what, but only when Tomasa died.

Dr. Madrid looked at the oldest child, Bartola. Eulalio wanted to keep Bartola. "Bartola can already make me a cup of coffee and cook," her father told Dr. Madrid.

"Well, I can't take any of the children now," Dr. Madrid said. She looked at eight-year-old Bartola, hair braided into a ponytail, wearing a tattered red gingham skirt and flip flops caked on the bottom with mud. Bartola spoke only when spoken to. She ran around the kitchen like a little woman fetching water, tending the fire, cooking tortillas, and brewing coffee. She ground corn in a grinder, washed dishes, and ran across the village with messages from her parents to neighbors. When Dr. Madrid caught a glimpse of Bartola's face, she looked worried, like she didn't really trust

Dr. Madrid, even though her mother had told her glowing things about the doctor and her home in Catacamas.

Dr. Madrid spent the night sleeping in a little church house near Eulalio's and Tomasa's house. The next morning, Bartola and her four-year-old sister, Fide, peeked into the window where the doctor was sleeping. Holding hands with her older sister, Fide's long hair was braided, pinned up in circles on the back of her head. She was barefooted and wore an orange dress with dingy beige lace. Dr. Madrid noticed a rash on Fide's face that looked like a burn—likely a reaction to a chemical in young mangoes or their stems that can cause a reaction much like poison ivy to the skin.

Fide followed Dr. Madrid the rest of the day. For Dr. Madrid this was a welcome sign that maybe the children could adjust to being with her until she found them a home with parents who wanted to adopt. Marcos was six years old and missing his front teeth, but smiled continually. He was wearing shorts, a green shirt, and rubber boots.

A few months passed and Tomasa died. After the funeral, Eulalio brought his four children to Dr. Madrid. The doctor was torn between the practicality of finding the children good homes and honoring Tomasa's request to keep them all together. She had been talking with a couple about the two-year-old boy, Wilito, and eventually Terry and Joni Stokes adopted him.

The doctor hoped to at least keep the other three siblings together. A North American in her fifties named Margo wanted to adopt the older three children. In order to give the children time to adjust, Dr. Madrid offered her home for Margo to stay with them. Having Margo and three children in the house for several transition months confirmed to Amanda that she herself was not the one to adopt the children. They behaved well, but the amount of care would be overwhelming when added to her responsibilities with Predisan.

After that transition period, when the children were settled with Margo, Dr. Madrid applied and was accepted to Loma Linda University in California. She moved to the United States for three years while she earned a doctorate in international public health with an emphasis on epidemiology and addictive behaviors.

In 1993, while completing her doctorate in the United States, she received a call from Honduras with the following news: Margo had been traveling with friends from Catacamas to Tegucigalpa; the children had stayed behind; because riding on the rough roads caused back pain for Margo, the driver had arranged a foam mattress in the covered pickup bed to allow Margo to recline; when the travelers arrived after a four hour drive, they opened the camper door and found Margo sleeping, but they could not wake her; they rushed her to the Tegucigalpa hospital, but she was brain dead on arrival.

They discovered that Margo had been breathing exhaust from the vehicle that was seeping into the unvented camper. Carbon monoxide poisoning had sent her into a coma. A week later, Margo died.

The children had lost two mothers in three years. The news of their adoptive mother's death shook the children, and their biological father, Eulalio, called Dr. Madrid.

"I'll take the children back where their feet will be in the mud," Eulalio said. He used a Spanish slang phrase that figuratively means living in poverty. Dr. Madrid told Eulalio that she would find a way to care for the children and that they need not return to "put their feet in the mud." Instead, missionaries Kent and Jamie Taylor took the children in until Dr. Madrid returned to Honduras.

When Dr. Madrid returned, she knew once again what she had to do. This time she felt God showing her that she had avoided the decision long enough. Dr. Madrid took the children into her home and began the protracted legal process of adopting Tomasa's and Eulalio's three children, Fide, 8, Marcos, 10, and Bartola, 12.

Amanda now faced life with three children to raise on her own. Her Predisan co-workers and other friends helped, but she took ultimate responsibility. She also resumed the role of directing Predisan after Doris Clark had filled in for three years in Amanda's absence. Many operational elements of Predisan changed for good while the doctor was away. But now Dr. Madrid had to understand new procedures as well as explore how to implement what she learned in public health, addiction, and epidemiology. Aware of this, Doris left on furlough in the United States for several months in order to give Dr. Madrid the space to again find her sea legs as captain of the Predisan ship.

Dr. Madrid had not married, and now her prospects of marrying or even dating had diminished by a factor of three. One day Eulalio came to speak with Dr. Madrid in Catacamas. His brow furrowed, and he hesitated to speak.

"Tell me, Eulalio, how are you doing on your own?" Dr. Madrid said.

He paused, letting the question settle in. "I've met a woman," Eulalio began. "She's a Christian."

Dr. Madrid tried to fill in the blanks. She understood he meant to marry the woman and that he was asking Amanda's permission. He seemed to Dr. Madrid more like the eldest brother of the children than their father. She felt as if she were talking to her son.

"Oh, that's good. Eulalio, you are a widowed man. You can get married again," Dr. Madrid said.

"But I don't know how to tell the children," Eulalio said.

Dr. Madrid thought, then said, "Don't worry, I'll tell them. They'll be fine, Eulalio. I think they will be happy for you."

Eulalio relaxed, took a deep breath. *"Yo no tengo el talento vivir solo.* I have realized I don't have the talent to live alone," Eulalio said.

Dr. Madrid laughed at Eulalio's way of describing his need for a wife: *No tengo el talento.*

Dr. Madrid wondered if *she* had that talent to live alone. So far she did, but it wasn't always a virtuoso performance.

She trained through books and acquaintances to be a good single mother. She embraced her own singleness, reading what Apostle Paul said in 1 Corinthians 7:34-35: "And the unmarried woman and the virgin are anxious about the affairs of the Lord, so that they may be holy in body and spirit; but the married woman is anxious about the affairs of the world, how to please her husband. I say this for your own benefit, not to put any restraint upon you, but to promote good order and unhindered devotion to the Lord."

She found this true of herself. In dating relationships, Amanda had learned that she became too dependent on the other person, and this stifled her devotion to God and to her work. In her forties and fifties she began to appreciate being single, the blessings, the freedom: completing medical school, working in mountain clinics, directing Predisan, opening CEREPA, traveling, consulting. It would have taken a very unique and liberal man to allow her to do so many of those things while married.

Through her years in Catacamas, however, the doctor continued to struggle with the social implications of being single. On the one hand, she felt her singleness gave young girls a positive role model—that one didn't have to be married to be valuable in society and to God. On the other hand, some men thought that since she was single she must be desperate for a man. If she ever detected this attitude in a man, she would not go out with him again.

Over time she realized that married women were often wary of her. They thought a single woman was ready to pounce on any man she could find, even if married. At parties where medical staff gathered, the doctor's wives sat close to their husbands, saying to Amanda with their eyes, *He's mine.*

The women were protective of their men for good reason but not necessarily because Amanda posed a threat. Many of those men would likely have an affair with her if she was willing, but she committed to celibacy until marriage. Even in villages women felt threatened. She learned that in order to have any reasonable contact with males, she often needed to make friends with the woman first to affirm that she was safe for friendship.

Before she adopted the three children, Maria Antonia pressured Amanda.

"I want you to bear grandchildren for me!"

"You already have forty grandchildren, Mama!" Amanda said. She had learned to rebuff the onslaught of advice about her life so she could find her own way.

Amanda didn't believe she had time to be married. First it was medical school, then serving in the military, practicing medicine, then moving to Catacamas—who would want to move there with her?—then founding a series of clinics, an addiction treatment center, and adopting children. Thoughts of marrying a man, however, still trailed behind her. But her life was going too fast for many men to accept.

After adopting the children, some people assumed she was a single biological mother of the children. In Honduras, as in many places in the world, there was a socially negative stigma of being a single mother.

When a group gathered at Dr. Madrid's house, one man saw photos of children throughout the house, but there were no photos of a father or husband. The man reasoned that her husband probably died, that they didn't want to have his picture visible. When Dr. Madrid sat for an interview to be considered as a board member of a Christian non-profit, the men seemed impressed with her skills and wanted her to be part of their board.

During the meeting, her status as a single mother came up, and an aura of judgment hung over the table.

"Do you have a husband," one board member inquired.

"No, I don't have a husband." No further explanation.

"Does the father of your kids see them often?" the same board member asked. "Yes, he does."

One of Dr. Madrid's grand reprisals on men was the joy of egging them on. She told the board the children's ages and made no reference to a husband, letting them think what they wanted to think—or stay curiously confused as she wanted them to be. They must have thought well enough of her, because they invited her to join the non-profit's board.

Some while later she became good friends with the board member who had asked her about a husband. Adoption was not very common in Honduras, so the idea hadn't entered the man's mind. He also didn't want to offend her by asking about a husband who may not be in the picture. Months later he asked her, "Why didn't you give it up and tell me?"

"Why didn't you just ask me directly?" Dr. Madrid shot back.

"Please forgive me," the man pleaded. "I also have to ask God to forgive me." Dr. Madrid didn't want to make light of the man's sincerity but she thought it was funny.

One Valentine's Day a man came to take Dr. Madrid out on a date. Fide, about ten at the time, put her hands on her hips and said, "You be home at nine o'clock, not a minute later."

"I'm the adult here!" Amanda said.

Upset and embarrassed, Fide ran into the girls' bedroom and slammed the door.

Amanda went to her door and whispered firmly, "Fide, open this door."

Fide opened the door, wanting to know, "Why do you not take us with you?"

"What are you afraid of, Fide?"

"That you are leaving us."

Amanda wrapped her hands around Fide's face, leaned down so she was looking directly in her eyes and said, "Fide, I will never leave you."

She told Fide a story about when she took her to play with a friend. "I did not stay, but you stayed with your friend. So I'm going with my friend, and you are not coming, just like I didn't stay with you when you played with your friend."

Amanda left with her friend, and during the date she thought about Fide the whole time. She wasn't sure how well the man reacted to Fide's fit. She told her children, "If I marry it will be someone who will want to 'marry' you too."

When Dr. Madrid paid bills, she would say, "This is the time of the month I would like to have a rich husband to pay all these bills." But when the children complained about the absence of such a man, Dr. Madrid would remind them, "There *is* a father in this house! *God* is the father in this house."

Marcos wanted a man around. One day he saw a man on the street whom they knew and he said to his mother, "He'd be a good man for you to marry."

"Yes, he would, but he smokes," Dr. Madrid said.

"Mama, you never said anything about smoking, but you need someone who has money, and he has money!"

She laughed but also felt pangs of guilt. Was she being self-ish for not settling down and marrying, even though she just couldn't accept a man who wasn't willing to go along with the adoption of three children and her intense work? So she invited their biological father, Eulalio, to visit as often as he was willing. She worked hard to connect the children with good male role models: the husband of the high school principal, the youth minister, and scout leaders.

In 1998, Amanda's sister, Elsita, learned in a medical checkup that her cancer had returned. She was in the hospital in Tegucigalpa. Dr. Madrid decided to take the children and visit Elsita. They drove in Dr. Madrid's Mitsubishi Montero the four-hour drive from Catacamas. On the return trip Dr. Madrid's oldest daughter, Bartola, who was seventeen, was driving on the highway near Juticalpa, halfway between Tegucigalpa and Catacamas. The road was smooth and wide in some places but narrow and potholed in others. In the mountain terrain, you might find a surprise around a bend or over a hill, perhaps a truck in your lane passing another slower vehicle.

In a flash, large cargo truck was too close, their vehicle was forced off the road, and Bartola lost control; the Montero SUV spun and rolled several times down an incline, settling in a ditch below the road. The driver's side roof above where Bartola sat was crushed like an aluminum can underfoot, but she was still inside the vehicle. They came to rest with the tires facing up, and the family all hanging upside down in their seats. They had worn their seatbelts. An eerie silence settled after they stopped rolling.

Amanda felt panic to know the condition of the children. She tried shaking off the dizziness but could barely move her neck. She yelled for each one to respond. Fide was crying in the back seat. That was a good sign. The roof was so badly caved in, she could not get a good view of Bartola, who assured her mother that she was alive; but there was great remorse and shock in her voice.

"Marcos!" Amanda called out. Nothing. He did not respond from the back seat. She couldn't see him.

"Marcos, do you hear me!?" She screamed.

"Marcos! Are you there!? Marcos!"

Was he thrown out of the car when it rolled!? Where was he?

Then Fide through her sobs assured the two in the front seat that Marcos was there, next to her. His silence frightened Amanda. She thought Marcos was dead.

Finally Marcos groaned. Amanda thanked God. Anything! Any noise would do. Her son was alive! The loss of control, the tumbling, the twisting of metal, hanging upside down. Through the entire horrific wreck, Marcos had slept.

Dr. Madrid felt lightheaded, the world spun, her children's voices sounded like echoes. She felt like fainting but she couldn't. Blacking out would mean she wouldn't be able to help the children with their injuries. She felt the tortuous sensation when you want to fall asleep but you know you cannot. Her neck hurt. The shock had masked the pain, but she knew something was terribly wrong. Strange sensations and throbbing pain in her arms signaled trouble.

Dr. Madrid was bleeding from a laceration on her head. She didn't know if it was dizziness, shock, or being upside down that made it seem impossible to move. Neighbors who heard the commotion and travelers from the road stopped their vehicles and ran down the embankment. Dr. Madrid managed to pull herself and the girls out of the vehicle before people arrived. But she realized that something serious had indeed happened to her, and she lay back in the grass.

People started to gather around. "Please do not touch me!" Dr. Madrid said. She could barely get the words out.

"Find my son first," she said. Dr. Madrid wanted the children taken safely away from the car. Would the car catch fire? Explode? Before the rescuers reached Marcos, he woke up, unbuckled his seat belt, and pulled himself out of a broken window.

Flat on her back, she asked each child to come closer so she could look into their pupils and at their lacerations. Each had a few scrapes and cuts but nothing that was bleeding badly. Dr. Madrid had a long gash on the left side of her head where she hit the windshield support bar. She bled heavily, so Bartola and Fide put pressure on the wound with a t-shirt, consoling their mother.

Among the rescuers, a man in his forties looked confident and inspired trust in Amanda. He said he wanted to get her to the hospital quickly.

"But I may have a spinal injury," Dr. Madrid said. "Can you get a piece of wood to keep me stable?" The man instructed a group of young men to run find a piece of wood about six feet long and at least a foot wide.

Struggling to stay conscious, Dr. Madrid asked the man to make a roll of clothes to keep her neck as stable as possible. No paramedics or ambulances would be available this far out of Tegucigalpa, and even in the capital city it was difficult to get an ambulance with medics for automobile accidents. The man said he had a small pickup and would transport her to the hospital in Juticalpa less than an hour away.

The young men returned with a long board and placed her carefully on it; then the man helped them carry the doctor to his pickup. The children gathered around her.

"Please, Mama! Please don't die!" Marcos said.

"You won't get rid of me this easily," Amanda said, slurring her words.

"Mama! Stop, please do not die, stay awake, Mama!" Fide and Bartola pleaded. Bartola was inconsolable.

"Listen all of you! I have NO plans to die!" But she *did* want to faint, sleep, anything.

The man drove the children and Dr. Madrid toward the hospital in Juticalpa.

*Please God, I'm begging you to keep me alive only for these children. They don't need another mother dying on them!*

Upon arrival at the hospital in Juticalpa, the man who drove them also made important calls from the hospital phone. Getting the numbers from the children, he called Amanda's mother, Maria Antonia, and co-workers, Paul and Katherine Evanson. The Evansons raced from Catacamas to Juticalpa to attend to Amanda and the children.

When Paul and Katherine arrived, Amanda's head had been bandaged, and the medical staff was preparing to x-ray her neck and spine. When the doctors assessed Dr. Madrid's injuries and told Amanda and the others, they all decided it would be best to stabilize and transfer her to the hospital in Tegucigalpa.

"Who was the man who called us?" Katherine asked.

"He found us right after the wreck. He saved our lives," Amanda said.

"Do you know his name?"

"No. He made sure my neck was stable, put me in the back of his pickup, drove us here," Amanda said. "He called you, then he left."

Was he an angel?

Dr. Madrid's inauspicious return to the Tegucigalpa hospital created a stir among the attending doctors who knew her, and she was given much attention and assessment. The next day Maria Antonia arrived from La Ceiba to help care for her. She and Katherine picked glass out of the children's and Amanda's hair. None of the children were badly injured, but something was not right with their mother. The doctor at the hospital in Tegucigalpa returned from looking at the x-rays with bad news.

Dr. Madrid's neck was broken.

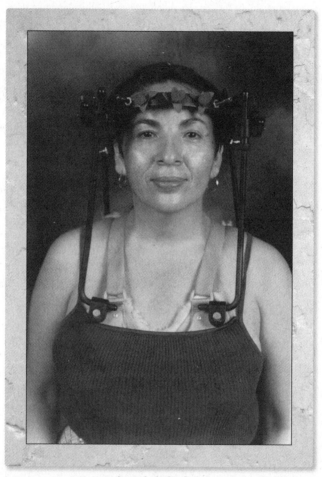

*Amanda in her halo.*

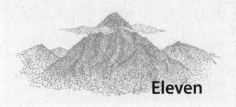

# Eleven

# THE HALO EFFECT

**The wreck broke Dr. Madrid's C4 and C5 vertebrae in her neck, partially paralyzing her.**

The doctors stabilized her, but she would need an apparatus to immobilize her neck and head. On a pain scale of one to ten, Amanda's ranged from seven to nine. For weeks after the wreck, Dr. Madrid was in traction and could not move her neck or leave the hospital bed. Then Paul Evanson called his cousin, Charlie Branch, chief of neurosurgery at Wake Forest, to come help. Dr. Branch flew to Honduras with three halo devices. He placed one of the circular steel devices around Dr. Madrid's head. Screws fit through holes in the steel band, then the screws were drilled into her skull. The halo included external supports leading to a shoulder and chest harness.

After a month and a half of recovery, the doctor began working from her hospital room, dictating letters, hearing from assistants about clinic issues and helping make decisions. She even signed a major medical grant contract for Predisan while in the hospital.

She also passed time during the eight-week hospital stay by reading the Bible and many other books. At the same hospital, a psychologist treated Bartola with therapy for the trauma and guilt she felt after the accident.

Follow up visits to the hospital and full recovery extended over the next year. After returning to Catacamas nearly two months after the accident, physical limitations restricted what Dr. Madrid could do. She even felt emotional energy in short supply. Before the wreck, every issue was a battle worth fighting for. She did not choose her battles well. During her recovery she learned that not every issue is worth fighting for or having her way.

Almost dying emotionally shook Dr. Madrid and the children. She didn't want Bartola to carry guilt for her mother's injuries. Fide and Bartola seemed traumatized by the wreck, quietly processing it in the months afterward. Fourteen-year-old Marcos bragged that he'd pulled himself out of the vehicle after the wreck. He and the girls had already seen two mothers die, and now they had faced the possibility of a third dying. Not wanting Bartola to resist driving the rest of her life for fear of another accident, Dr. Madrid bought her oldest daughter a small car.

Dr. Madrid was not afraid to die, but her worst fear was the thought of leaving the children. During the ordeal, Elsita's face continued to appear in Amanda's mind's eye. She knew her sister was close to death.

Amanda was still in her halo when her sister died of cancer. She attended Elsita's funeral in her halo. The continuing pain along her spine, the grief, and the stress of relying on others because of immobility all weighed heavily on Amanda. Overwhelmed with things she could not control, she latched on to a few things she could control.

As the day of Marcos's fifteenth birthday approached, Dr. Madrid had an idea to throw a big party for him, like the *Quinceañeras* but a masculine version.

*Quinceañeras* are the rite of passage for fifteen-year-old girls in Latin American cultures. Catholics celebrate *Quinceañeras* with religious significance around a mass, but culturally there are many who throw parties with little reference to the church or faith. Often the family buys their daughter a new dress, sometimes pink or white to show purity, and the girl dances with her father. The family gives the fifteen-year-old girl a tiara to signify her importance in the family as a princess. Family and friends dress up to celebrate this rite of passage into womanhood.

Dr. Madrid believed boys also ought to have a more genuine rite of passage, a big celebration; but such a celebration is uncommon in Latin American culture. Instead, boys are often led into adulthood by men who get the boys drunk for the first time, take them to see a stripper or even a prostitute. Those same boys attend *Quinceañeras* often with a decidedly more perverse view of womanhood than the purity rites they witness.

Dr. Madrid wanted to set out a godly and morally pure path for Marcos, making it clear that he would not participate in the perverse rites of passage that many boys experienced. Though she was in no shape to throw a party for Marcos, she wanted to do something.

In the closing days of October 1998, with Hurricane Mitch swirling over the Bay Islands along the north coast of Honduras, Dr. Madrid enlisted the help of her daughters, the church, and other friends to plan a fifteenth birthday party for Marcos.

Then Hurricane Mitch made landfall. The storm sat on top of Honduras as a tropical depression between October 27 and October 31, dumping thirty-five inches of rain in some regions of the country. Rivers swelled, flooding thousands of homes and businesses in rural and urban areas. In Tegucigalpa floods and mudslides toppled house upon house, people were drowned, buried alive, swept away by the rivers flowing through the streets.

Hurricane Mitch claimed 9,086 lives across Central America and 5,677 of those deaths were in Honduras. Mitch was one of the five worst hurricanes since records have been kept from the late 1800s. An estimated 70,000 homes were damaged, ninety-two bridges were washed out or damaged, and electricity and water services were down for months.

While people suffered, Dr. Madrid remained in her halo. The apparatus that immobilized her neck prevented the doctor from doing what she wanted to do: help the victims of Hurricane Mitch. One of the areas around the halo became infected. She wanted it off her head, the screws out, the support off her shoulders. The holes hurt more than her neck now. It was time to take it off. Whose permission did she need anyway? She was a doctor. She knew her own body. Nobody could tell her no.

She asked her friend, Katherine, to help her remove the halo. The doctor took deep breaths, and told Katherine to work quickly. Katherine unscrewed the pins of the halo that were sunk into the doctor's skin and skull. Amanda closed her eyes, gritted her teeth, and felt like fainting—the way she felt the day of the wreck.

When the last pin was unscrewed, she was free. Katherine applied antibiotic ointment and bandages. Dr. Madrid moved her neck slightly in different directions. The muscles had atrophied. Most neck-injured patients needed rest and weeks of physical therapy before doing anything strenuous. The day the halo came off, however, Dr. Madrid insisted on going to a site where people were being housed after Hurricane Mitch, where victims needed medical attention.

Katherine dropped the halo on the kitchen table with a thunk; she attached a simple foam brace to the doctor's neck and drove her to the Catholic Church, which provided its retreat center dormitory in Catacamas to house storm victims.

Over the next few weeks, the doctor organized efforts to feed hundreds and performed triage and mobile care for patients needing immediate care. She instructed volunteers and Predisan staff to collect clothing and bedding for families that lost everything in the flood. With other volunteers, the doctor cleaned toilets at the dormitory, doing what they could to slow or stop the spread of cholera.

After ensuring that all who needed temporary housing were cared for, she and local leaders turned to long-term efforts to raise money, find land, and rebuild permanent housing. Aid poured in from private and government sources worldwide.

While the doctor helped storm victims, it seemed Hurricane Mitch was healing Dr. Madrid, putting her back on her feet, curbing her depression. Marcos's *Quinceañero*—Dr. Madrid made up this masculine form for a fifteen-year-old's rite of passage—was still in the back of her mind as she served storm victims. Weeks after Hurricane Mitch, Dr. Madrid enacted her own subdued version of a *Quinceañero* for Marcos. She baked cinnamon rolls, lit a candle for Marcos to blow out, and the family of four enjoyed an intimate meal that reminded them all how grateful they were to be alive and together after the wreck and storm.

Hurricane Mitch continued to impact Honduras for many years. Mitch put his imprint on Predisan as well. For years the Good Samaritan Clinic served the wide range of needs of a community that suffered loss of life, homes, and jobs. Predisan raised grant money for, then planned, contracted, and managed the construction of a new housing district. Partnering with the city of Catacamas, the Lions Club, Catholic Church, Holiness Church, and El Sembrador Ministry, Predisan also coordinated and funded construction of a clean water and sanitation system for the new neighborhood. The Good Samaritan Clinic became a center of outreach to a devastated population. Much of the funding to build a larger clinic that would serve more people came through private donations or grants from the governments of the United States and Honduras.

Some who began working for Predisan after Mitch continued with the organization. Keydy Flores began in 1998 as an intern, but she stayed on and eventually became an assistant director as Dr. Madrid's right arm, staying at the office with the doctor till late hours or reporting to the doctor's house Saturday mornings to finish an urgent project.

New needs after Hurricane Mitch created a leadership vacuum that Dr. Madrid filled. Her life had prepared her for growing Predisan into a larger organization. She now possessed the skills to lead a bigger organization than a clinic run out of a rented house.

Dr. Madrid—with all her contacts in Tegucigalpa, from university, medical school, military, and government—was active and influential in helping Predisan apply for and receive grant aid. With the new funding, Predisan diligently developed new programs that benefited both the country and Predisan's mission in the mountains. For example, at a time when nurses were needed in the mountains, and most did not want to leave their families to live there, Dr. Madrid approached the government with a proposal to train health care workers. Half would work in Predisan clinics, half in government health care.

More health care workers were needed in the mountain clinics to deliver babies. Traditionally, women gave birth at home or in a midwife's house. According to newer Honduran health codes, however, midwives or Traditional Birth Assistants (TBA) could no longer practice in their own homes.

TBA Doña Carmen had delivered hundreds of babies in the mountains near one of Predisan's rural clinics. A plump and imposing woman in her fifties, Doña Carmen's house was nestled in a ravine next to the dirt road that followed the ridgelines of the mountain. Banana plants on the slopes surrounding Doña Carmen's house leaned over with the weight of the green stalks of bananas large as five gallon buckets.

Doña Carmen had an extra room in her house where women came to stay during the last weeks of their pregnancy. Childbearing women loved Doña Carmen because she attended to their needs at this crucial time in their lives, in ways no one else in that region ever did. Women would rather go to Doña Carmen's house than to a sterile medical clinic or hospital in town.

Dr. Madrid offered free training for Doña Carmen, but she refused. Doña Carmen's mother and her grandmother were TBAs, and she learned from them how to identify at-risk patients by physical examination, not by ultrasound.

Superstition also holds some women back from going to clinics and hospitals. When a baby or mother dies in the hospital, people often say it's the doctor's fault. When a baby or mother dies in a TBA's care, people might say it's the cycle of the moon or something in nature that caused the death.

When a baby boy is born, a TBA says to the mother, "You win the hen." For the birth of a boy, she says the mother deserves a delicacy of homemade chicken soup. For the birth of a girl, in contrast, the TBA offers a corn tortilla with cheese as a consolation. A TBA charges more money for her services if the baby is a boy—2,000 lempiras, $100, or two weeks wages for an average Honduran; but if she delivers a baby girl, the TBA asks for 1,000 lempiras, $50, or one week's wages.

Gender inequality was a stagnant pond Amanda had to swim in her whole life. Though Dr. Madrid earned multiple degrees and developed leadership qualities, in Honduras she still faced gender inequality and discrimination. Inequality did not stop when she became a doctor, a military medical officer, and eventually the executive director of one of the largest non-profit organizations in Honduras.

A new millennium was approaching but it seemed to Amanda as if she were living in the dark ages when a group of twenty men organized to oust her from her position of executive director of Predisan. The men wrote a letter to a Predisan-funding church in the United States, asking for Dr. Madrid's removal as executive director.

The first issue, they said, was that Dr. Madrid was a woman. They didn't think a woman ought to run an organization as influential as Predisan. She had also started preaching in the local church, and these men were of the mind that women were not to speak in church.

The group's second issue was money. Government grants, they said, would help Predisan do medical work, but they reasoned that government funds would legally prevent the organization from doing half of its mission: the "preach" part of "to preach and to heal" would be restricted by government involvement.

"This government money is evil and will prevent us from doing God's work," one of the men said to Dr. Madrid.

"The devil wants to use money for his own pleasure," Dr. Madrid told the church member, "but God trains us to use money for his purposes. We don't have the law requiring strict separation of church and state here like they do in the United States."

The group's third and final issue was about personnel in Predisan. As the Good Samaritan Clinic, CEREPA, and outpost clinics grew, Dr. Madrid hired more and more qualified medical personnel. The group of men wanted the doctor to hire only people from their denomination. Dr. Madrid protested that not enough qualified medical workers were also members of their church. So Dr. Madrid hired qualified medical workers who were good people—nearly all professing Christians—regardless of their church affiliation.

Dr. Madrid's critics said she shouldn't be vocal and preach, yet they criticized her and Predisan for not preaching enough, for focusing too much on the medical side of the organization. The letter concluded that the men were "cancelling" Dr. Madrid's privilege to teach and preach in their church.

She would not be stopped from speaking about Jesus wherever she was. In her medical work, Dr. Madrid had many opportunities to show the love of God and to share the story of Jesus. Not only that, but she also did not hesitate to tell government officials or anyone else—from *campesinos* to consulars—about Jesus.

One day a professor directing an institute for alcohol addiction asked Dr. Madrid, "What are you doing in Olancho?"

"God called me to work there with people with addictions."

"Hmmm, interesting. A religious group working with serious social problems. I wonder why that is?" the professor asked.

"It's because we love God," Dr. Madrid said.

The professor was accustomed to philosophical answers, even from clergy. The directness of her answer seemed to startle the professor. He didn't know what to do with it, so he begged off the conversation, holding up a hand.

"Maybe another time you can tell me more about that," he said. "I have another appointment."

"I'll be happy to," Dr. Madrid replied.

On a subsequent visit to the professor's office, Dr. Madrid took a copy of the Bible. She explained her faith in God with scriptures she read aloud. The professor said he would not likely come to a church, but he quietly listened to Dr. Madrid tell him the gospel of grace, love, and hope in Christ. Then she prayed for the professor and left.

Meanwhile, the letter of critique from the twenty Honduran church leaders reached the supporting church in the United States. She would have to make a trip to Atlanta, Georgia to defend herself and Predisan from the attack of her own countrymen.

Amanda hoped her supporting church would indeed support her, but she had not fully discussed these issues about gender equality and leadership with the mission committee in Atlanta. She did not know what the members thought or how they would react. Would they side with the Honduran group who'd sent the letter? She began forming her resignation speech to the board in case they sided with her critics.

Amanda felt as if she were a girl again in La Jigua being sent to the principal's office. What had she done wrong? She had work to do in the clinics. Why had she left the Pentecostal church of her childhood where she could speak freely and entered a close-minded church like this?

It was becoming clear, however, that this was indeed a denomination with traditions and mores that men and some women believed must be upheld at all costs. Some seemed to hold more tightly to tenets of the denomination passed on by missionaries than to Christ's words. This deeply disturbed Dr. Madrid. She strapped on her guns and readied herself for a fight.

In Tegucigalpa, when her brother had returned from a preaching school, he had convinced her that his denomination was the "one true church." In the 1980s, Amanda had seen how this church sought truth in the Bible only, wanted to be called "Christians only," and claimed no denominational affiliation. Her brothers had even convinced her to be re-baptized for the forgiveness of sins, because they told her the baptism she received at age fourteen in the Cangrejal River in La Ceiba was not valid. She was immersed, they said, for a witness to the church that she was a follower of

Christ, but if they didn't say they baptized her for the forgiveness of sins when she was fourteen, she needed to do it again.

She agreed back in Tegucigalpa to be re-baptized, but now in this baptism of fiery critique she regretted entering this particular church. Still, this was the church where she met the Clarks, that helped her start CEREPA, that helped her live her dream since she was a little girl to love and serve God the rest of her life as a doctor.

Not all Hondurans agreed with the group of twenty Honduran men. A sixty-two-year-old rancher and restaurant owner told a Predisan supporter that Dr. Madrid had given her life for the Honduran people. He said he didn't know how she accomplished all that she did, but he believed the doctor ought to continue using her God-given abilities to lead and to speak out.

"Dr. Madrid teaches and gives me good advice. I respect both her and the organization she directs, because she's a good example of helping poor people," the Honduran rancher said.

Dr. Madrid knew that many Hondurans supported her, and that comforted her. Yet the circular reasoning of detractors gnawed on her confidence and joy. They didn't want her to preach in the church or publicly because she was a woman, and yet some of the same men criticized her because she and Predisan were not preaching enough.

The mission committee of the Atlanta church asked Dr. Madrid many questions.

"What are your main beliefs?"

Dr. Madrid explained she believed in the church as the body of Christ's followers, that the main work of the church is sharing the love of God.

"What's your motivation for working with Predisan?" one member of the committee asked.

Dr. Madrid wanted to be snarky, but she gritted her teeth and remained respectful. The mission committee of the Atlanta church did their job to ascertain what the problem was and to see that the work of Predisan continued. The committee leader showed Dr. Madrid the letter that the Honduran preachers had written.

As she read the letter she trembled, her chest tightened, and her heart raced. Some of those men had been her close friends for many years. They called each other brother and sister in Christ.

The long letter said the Honduran church leaders were forbidding Dr. Madrid from speaking in the church, because they said men—not women—are the God-ordained leaders of the church. This was the way of the Catholic Church, the way of many Evangelical churches, and now it had come down to this in her church. Women could teach other women or children. Women just couldn't lead other men, because men were the ones in authority over women.

She had given her life to serve God and the people of Olancho. So this was the conclusion of her Honduran brothers: that she was bad for Predisan, that she ought to be silent in the church? But then they blamed her for not preaching more at Predisan!?

"I don't believe a church is defined by whether or not women can lead," Dr. Madrid said. "If you want me to not lead because I'm a woman, you can fire me now. I'll go somewhere else," she told the committee.

A Predisan board member, Justin Myrick, had come to the meeting to support Dr. Madrid against the arguments of the Honduran church leaders. He had been instrumental in helping Predisan set up the health care system. He did not come to speak for a church but specifically to support Dr. Madrid and to carry on the work of Predisan.

Justin told Dr. Madrid that some people in Christian non-profits, universities, and ministries supported by a particular church tend to go with the flow—not rock the boat or buck the system—because to do otherwise might negatively impact their funding. For the sake of this leadership issue, was she willing to lose the support of Honduran Christian leaders and possibly a large supporting church in America? Was she jeopardizing the future support of Predisan?

"Keep doing what you are doing, Dr. Madrid," Justin Myrick said, smiling. "We need people like you." He explained that the Predisan board supported her leadership to preach and to heal. As for her local church involvement, Justin said, "Follow what your church leaders decide or find another church." As far as he and the board were concerned, Dr. Madrid's work with Predisan should continue without further interruption.

Then Justin added a parting word of wisdom. "Amanda, holster your guns." Dr. Madrid took a deep breath, sighed, then relaxed her shoulders and tried to smile. How could she go back to Honduras and lay down her guns when these Honduran men were so wrong?

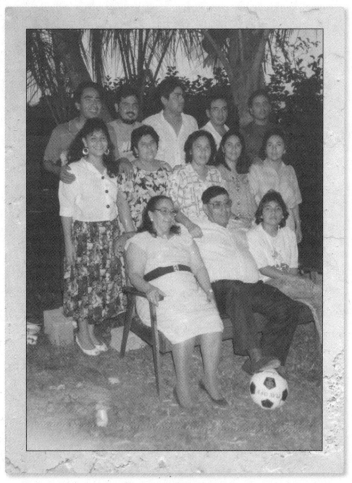

*Florencio's fútbol team.*

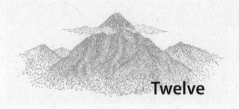

## Twelve

# LAY DOWN YOUR GUNS

**Amanda knew Justin Myrick was right, that she ought to lay down her guns, but she thought that would mean leaving her church that had "cancelled her privileges to** teach and preach." How could she remain silent? To Amanda, silent mostly meant passive. Did she need to lead in a more "lady-like" way? That thought infuriated her. She was trained to lead, not melt into the furniture. She would neither conform to male dominance nor would she agree that this was some sort of feminist agenda she pushed. If she stayed, she knew she would have to speak out—and preach the gospel. She felt strongly that she should leave. What else is a leader like her to do? Sit idly listening to the men who had rejected her as a leader? It seemed impossible for her to do. She had to leave.

But leaving posed a problem, since Predisan had been founded in this denomination with support from these churches in the United States and Honduras. What would happen if she left and went to another church? How would it impact local Predisan work? How would leaving impact her children? Bartola, Fide, and Marcos were teenagers who enjoyed the church's youth fellowship.

Amanda called the family together in their home.

"We need to leave our church," Amanda told her children.

"What? No! What about us and what we want?"

Her teenagers had friends in the church and had not felt the stabbing rejection Amanda had experienced.

"We don't want to leave. This is our church."

Amanda faced a difficult decision, so she asked the children for more time to think, to pray about what they must do.

During the crisis over her Predisan leadership, Amanda often woke at 3 a.m. to pray about next steps to take as a family. In her morning prayer sessions, she thought about how her children needed strong male role models. Through the years, many at the church had taken her children under their wings. Predisan remained very connected to her church, and the rural churches worked hand in hand with the mountain clinics. The church really had become part of her and her children's identities.

Amanda felt as if her heart was a sponge full of bitterness that God needed to wring out. One morning in prayer she felt as if she heard the whisper of the Holy Spirit telling her to stay, that there was another way. The anger and bitterness flowed out and a solution flowed in.

At the dinner table that night, Amanda announced to her children the conclusion she had come to in her prayer that morning.

"I'll teach the youth in our church," Amanda told her children. The twenty men who signed the letter were only prohibiting Amanda to teach and have authority over men. They had not cancelled her privileges to teach women and youth.

The children smiled—they liked the idea. They would do anything to stay with friends and a youth leader they loved—even if their mother had to become one of their youth leaders.

So Dr. Madrid stayed in the church that had "cancelled her privilege to preach." The church men deemed teaching teenagers "scriptural," since she would not be exercising authority over men. Dr. Madrid spoke to the current youth worker, asking if she could help. He was happy to have her assistance, so she began teaching and mentoring teenagers.

That Christmas Amanda went door to door, to the homes of all the church's children and teenagers. She wore a festive hat and gave them gifts of fresh fruit. Through the years, when someone in the church had a birthday, the doctor gathered a band of youth and adults to wake the person up at their house with a rousing rendition of *Feliz Cumpleaños* Happy Birthday.

One rainy day the youth had gathered at the church to play games. They moved a ping pong table indoors so they could play and not get wet. Later, when a church leader heard about the youth playing games in the church building, he scolded Dr. Madrid for bringing the game table into the church. Didn't she know it was wrong to play ping pong in the house of prayer? On another occasion Amanda was criticized for not disciplining teenagers who laughed during a prayer.

Amanda could not understand why people made issues out of small things but ignored huge problems in society like poverty, health care, and preaching the hope and love of Jesus Christ. Some wanted a "perfect" church, to have the "right" liturgy, but she realized that many churches did not teach practical ways to love others.

Just as the conflict in the church faded, family conflict put Amanda right back into the middle of the eleven. "These eleven children are my *fútbol* team," Florencio, Sr. often joked. But Florencio, Sr. seemed oblivious to the disunity on his *fútbol* team. Sometimes they played well together, but even as adult siblings, in 2003 the *fútbol* team faltered when their coach became deathly ill.

Amanda traveled from Tegucigalpa to La Ceiba when she received news of her father's acute sickness. She joined her mother, Maria Antonia, in caring for Florencio, Sr. When his health continued to spiral downward, his wife and daughter-turned-doctor decided to take Florencio to Tegucigalpa to admit him to the army hospital.

In the hospital bed, Florencio told Amanda that the reason he did not support her to enter medical school was because he did not want anything bad to happen to his Mayan Princess in the big city of Tegucigalpa. Amanda was unsure how to feel about this revelation. What he intended perhaps as a confession felt to Amanda like a slap in the face. So her father withheld his blessing so long because he feared for her safety?

After two weeks of illness, Florencio, Sr. died in the army hospital in Tegucigalpa. His body was transported back to La Ceiba where the family buried him on family land.

Soon after Florencio's death, the family grieved but did not quarrel; then questions arose about how Maria Antonia would receive and use the inheritance money. By Honduran standards Florencio, Sr. had done well financially, wisely planting crops, raising livestock, and employing workers to help him produce cash crops on his farm. While it was difficult to say directly, some of the siblings began to wonder if any of the inheritance would be given to them. What happens to the estate when Maria Antonia dies? Did she have a will? How would she divide everything among eleven children?

The Madrid family, like families in many cultures, found that discussing inheritance led to conflict. There were sentences prefaced with, "It would only be fair," and ended with, "I just want to make sure Mama is cared for, that's all."

A power struggle began in earnest by the first anniversary of the Madrid patriarch's death. Siblings stopped talking to one another, which perplexed Amanda. They'd all grown up with the same values in a Christian home. Why were they clamming up, taking sides, and allowing possessions and money to divide them?

As a result, five siblings aligned with their mother on several key issues related to the inheritance, and five were opposed. With Elsita deceased, now there was a five to five split, with Amanda joining one of the sides. When Florencio, Sr. died, the dam holding back the family feud broke and flooded the Madrid homes. Amanda saw herself as the family fixer, squarely in the middle, a mediator for all. Somehow even with the mistakes Florencio, Sr. had made, he held the family together, and Amanda wanted to do the same.

She'd heard about families dividing over inheritance issues, but she had believed her family to be the exception. They would never split over money and inheritance issues! How could this happen to her family? Money had always been important to Florencio and to Maria Antonia's mother-in-law, Tula, who had said about her children, *"Vivos para el pisto.* They are all smart to make money."* Now the inheritance, being smart to make money, did not seem like such a great value to possess.

The siblings hired attorneys and chose sides. Hatred was expressed and wounds opened. Dr. Madrid positioned herself where she perceived her skills could do the most good—in the middle of the conflict—but this stance was not considered neutral by her siblings. She was vilified on both sides of the family feud.

During this time Dr. Madrid left Honduras and Predisan to serve as a visiting professor at Oklahoma Christian University in Edmond, Oklahoma, from 2006-08 while her children attended school there. At the university she taught Spanish, Bible, Missions, and Community Health. Her research, speaking, and consulting brought a welcome reprieve from the family feud, the stress of her medical practice in Honduras, and the management of Predisan.

She traveled widely to consult in public health issues in Costa Rica, El Salvador, Guatemala, Nicaragua, Cuba, Kenya, England, France, Switzerland, Germany, Belgium, the Netherlands, North and South Korea, Mexico, Tanzania, Thailand, Indonesia, Peru, Panama, South Africa, and the United States. In her consultations she also observed successful methods in those countries, then returned to Honduras with new ideas for Predisan.

Her travels had put distance between her and the rancor of the family jockeying for position with their mother. When she returned to Honduras, however, the family strife washed over her again. She had begun building a new house in Catacamas, but when family conflict flared up, she wanted to abandon the building project, move to Tegucigalpa, hire a battalion of attorneys, and fight her siblings. She wanted to pick up her guns, this time in the war of "Who Loves Mom More." They were hurting Maria Antonia, and she would stand up for her mother. But the other siblings also claimed to love their mother.

Then, finally, she talked to her confidante and co-worker, Doris Clark. Doris assured Amanda that life is not always fair, and that what is required in every situation, particularly when it comes to such vitriol in a family, is love, forgiveness, and mercy.

After that conversation with Doris, Amanda decided that both groups were doing wrong. Her sister—on her side—wanted them to say things in court that were false. Amanda had never wanted the feud to go to court, and certainly now she wasn't going to perjure herself. She told her sister she was not going to say anything false in court, that with God's help she would hold to her values. She said her goal was to help her mother in the closing years of her life. She did not move to Tegucigalpa or hire a team of lawyers. What shocked the family most, however, was what she did next.

"I renounce my rights to any of the money that may come to the brothers and sisters," she told them.

This stance resolved her own emotional turmoil, but it did not resolve anything with her brothers and sisters. Now she was not on either side. She was once again in the middle. On both sides they said, "You are against us" and "You're trying to pretend you are a Christian and act holier than thou."

Those words sliced new cuts in Dr. Madrid's heart. She continued to pray for the whole situation more than anything else in life, though she didn't see a favorable outcome. The litigation continued.

Over time Dr. Madrid talked to all of her brothers and sisters, expressing her love for them, her disinterest in the money, and her desire for a renewed relationship while their mother was still living. Elder was simply not interested in reconciling. She told her recalcitrant brother that at least he could go see their mother to make the relationship right while she was still living, but his answer was cold: he had nothing to forgive her for; he had done nothing for which to be forgiven.

Maria Antonia suffered through the years of family war, grieved that her family was crumbling, like over-baked adobe bricks, and she didn't know what to do about it. Dr. Madrid became her communication proxy, but at least half of the siblings disregarded what Amanda had to say.

In 2008, Dr. Madrid moved Maria Antonia from La Ceiba to the doctor's home in Catacamas. Florencio's death and the family split had aged Maria Antonia rapidly. She developed Alzheimer's during these years living in her daughter's house, but this was one case of Alzheimer's that seemed to benefit the patient in an important way. She seemed to forget details of the current family problems, reveling instead in memories from her life with Florencio, Sr. and when the children were young. Even the family troubles they faced in Copán seemed to fade away, and her memories centered on the joyous times they shared, not the bitterness or pain.

In those years of living together, Dr. Madrid remembered the little prayer and birthing room in their house in Copán. Just as in those days, so Maria Antonia late in life continued to wake early in the morning to read the Bible and pray for her children. She didn't care as much about the material possessions as she cared about her children living in peace with one another.

One day Maria Antonia was lying on the couch in Dr. Madrid's house and she said to no one in particular: "I have everything I need here. I always wanted to have lots of flowers and birds." Dr. Madrid had parrots and flowers, and the calming beauty of the birds and flowers, soothed Maria Antonia in ways that Amanda had been comforted by the prayer room in her childhood home.

This vision of Maria Antonia's desire for peace made her want to help others get this kind of peace. What if she could teach others to lay down their guns of conflict? She herself had learned in a variety of settings to lay down her guns.

She read the book, *Crucial Conversations: Tools for Talking When Stakes are High*. What sets true leaders apart, the authors say, is their ability to have crucial conversations at the right time with the right people. Dr. Madrid bought copies of the book in Spanish and English for herself and her Predisan managers. Somewhere between raw aggression and passivity there was a better way to communicate, and she was determined to help Hondurans learn this better way. She and the Predisan board invited professionals in the field of conflict transformation to develop programs to help Hondurans at work, home, and church transform conflict and hatred into better communication.

Though others led the way in conflict transformation at Predisan, Amanda increasingly realized her destiny to be a person in the middle. She often found herself in the center of conflicts in her family, churches, clinics, and in the mountains. She held her ground firmly between passivity and violence, seeking solutions that transform lives. She was stubborn enough to believe that the attempt should still be made to reconcile, even among those who refused to consider reconciliation.

Dr. Madrid's life and Predisan had become focused on healing people holistically: spiritually, physically, and emotionally. She knew from her Bible reading that James 5:16 (NIV) says, "Therefore confess your sins to each other and pray for each other so that you may be healed." She desperately wanted to be healed and to help others heal. That had become the mission of her life: to preach and to heal.

At the end of 2011, Maria Antonia wanted to go home to La Ceiba. Amanda sensed this was her way of saying good bye to the other children. During Christmas Maria Antonia became ill. During a brief stay in the hospital, Amanda treated Maria Antonia, but she died New Year's Eve 2011.

Amanda had watched her mother get up early each morning to pray for her family. Give her a place to pray, birds singing, flowers, and children who love one another—who were not arguing or suing one another—and she was happy. Amanda thought her mother's Alzheimer's was a blessing at the end of her life, because she seemed no longer bothered by the protracted family conflict between Florencio's death in 2003 and Maria Antonia's death in 2011.

Instead Maria Antonia remembered the distant memories of the farm in Copán, giving birth to eleven children, the reunion of her family at Christmas in 1964 in El Cacao outside La Ceiba, and the day Amanda became a doctor. Maria Antonia had for years introduced her adult daughter as *"Mi hija la doctora.* My daughter the doctor."

Dr. Madrid read a lot about grief, psychology, and families. While this helped her cope with loss, no amount of reading seemed to give her lasting peace. Amanda believed the three years Maria Antonia lived with her were a gift from God. Maria Antonia had been like a giant *Ceiba* tree in the forest of Dr. Madrid's life, always there. Even with Alzheimer's and able to do little to help Amanda, Maria Antonia gave her daughter a presence of stability and emotional support.

Dr. Madrid read a book titled, *Heaven,* by Randy Alcorn, and some vital ideas surfaced for her about life and death, that death marks a gateway into a new eternal reality for the follower of Christ, an immortality that is not gifted to every human but given alone through belief in the resurrected Christ. The book encouraged her to keep living a fruitful life that is also a preparation for the life to come.

At Maria Antonia's funeral, the family splintered further, and Dr. Madrid's two younger sisters did not speak to Amanda or even look at her. Even the next generation of grandchildren had split about whether or not they ought to come to the funeral, because they hated the family war, and the funeral was no place to fight that war. Some even suggested that Maria Antonia's children who were unsupportive of her were unworthy to attend her funeral.

Two nieces who were close to Dr. Madrid stood by her side, even when their mothers were estranged from Amanda. Co-workers from Predisan traveled to La Ceiba to share their leader's grief. Predisan had its share of conflicts. She had to fire people who mistreated employees, embezzled money, or had affairs. Predisan, like her family, was an organization full of imperfect people, including herself. Tears flowed when the doctor saw her Predisan friends enter the church for the funeral, and she fell into their arms, because the Predisan family was bonded in a way her own family was not.

After the funeral, Amanda visited one of her sisters in La Ceiba. When she left her sister's house, she felt a catharsis but also emptiness. Losing Maria Antonia felt like losing a spouse she never had.

She would be returning to Catacamas and an empty house.

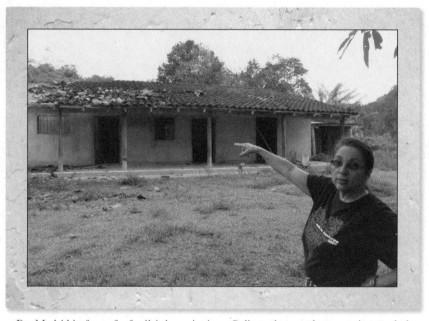

*Dr. Madrid in front of a family's house in Agua Caliente that cartel mercenaries attacked.*

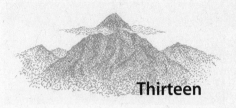

# Thirteen

# HIGH HEELS AND COMBAT BOOTS

**When a child's parents both die, the world calls them an orphan, signaling their need for compassion and care. When an adult loses both parents, however, the world** has no label or special operating instructions. But something inexplicable happens when anyone, particularly a single person, loses both parents. Amanda did not feel she had totally lost the mainsails on her ship, but for a season she felt becalmed—without wind to fill them. Siblings remained distant, Maria Antonia no longer watched birds through Amanda's windows, and the house felt cavernous and filled with echoes when she talked on the phone.

Sibling conflict compounded the loss of Maria Antonia and Florencio, Sr. The family ordeal and loss gave way to a shift in Amanda's identity as daughter and adoptive mother to *abuela*. Two years before Maria Antonia's death, Dr. Madrid had become a grandmother when her son, Marcos, and daughter-in-law, Rebekah, had a baby named Leyla. For a woman who wasn't married yet, who adopted three children and put them all through college, having a grandchild sent a rush of adrenaline through her veins that if bottled could fuel a rocket to Mars.

She would not live alone for long. Soon after Maria Antonia's death, Dr. Madrid's oldest daughter, Bartola, engaged and nearing her thirties, came to live with Amanda in her house in Catacamas. Her daughter, Fide, married and moved with her husband to Europe.

Marcos and Rebekah lived in Catacamas, where Marcos managed a coffee plantation in the mountains higher up from the network of mountain clinics in the Cuyamel River Valley. Where Marcos planted a cash crop for local Hondurans to benefit with jobs and industry, others were trafficking drugs through the same region. Amanda feared for the lives of her son, daughter-in-law, and granddaughter.

Amanda's nephew Roger, also a doctor, was like a son to her. Roger and his wife had a baby boy, David, in late 2012. Amanda counted David as one of her grandchildren. Rebekah gave birth in early 2013 to a boy, Jonathan.

Amanda could have wrung her hands about the safety of her children and grandchildren. She could have settled on a hill like her grandmother Tula, watching over her brood. She could have fought for a family farm for the next generation like Maria Antonia; but Amanda chose another battle in the beginning of her years as *Abuela.*

In her mid-fifties, she made a series of decisions few grandmothers would make. What she had learned about conflict and her desire to see people living at peace, influenced her decisions deeply. After what happened between 2009 to 2011, she believed she truly had no choice but to act decisively. During those two years, in the mountains near Predisan clinics, forty-two murders had been committed due to the explosive mix of drugs, guns, and great envy.

Dr. Madrid received news of one terrible massacre in the mountain villages, where a four-year-old boy named Juan had been brought into the clinic in Agua Caliente. Juan had been caught in crossfire during a turf battle between two local families—one family strongly connected to drug traffickers, the other family rising up against the traffickers' attempted control of the village.

One of the groups ambushed the other at the home of Juan's grandparents. Attackers bullets hit four-year-old Juan's leg. Juan's father and grandmother attempted to defend their family, mortally wounding several of the attackers before both Juan's father and grandmother were shot.

Four-year-old Juan had an eight-year-old brother who stayed by his younger brother's side. He took off his shirt and wrapped it tightly around Juan's leg to stop the bleeding. He quieted his bleeding brother so attackers would not hear them, but they needed help. Hours passed, flies gathered around the corpses outside and in the doorways or windows of the house, vultures circled overhead, and fear and confusion overcame the neighbors. Juan remained in the house with his brother but without medical care. Their six-year-old sister alternately ran and hid for hours until she found a house in another village in which to take refuge.

News of the battle reached clinic headquarters, CEDECO, saying survivors from the gun battle needed medical care. Frank Lopez, a heavy-set man in his forties who had grown up in the Cuyamel River Valley and knew the feuding families, many of whom were his schoolmates and cousins, formed a rescue team. Frank's uncle and father, two nurses, and several neighbors accompanied Frank. When they arrived at the scene of the battle, they found six badly wounded with spiking fevers; they administered IVs, started antibiotics, and wrapped wounds to stop the bleeding. Without the medical team, all six would likely have died. All six survived. Nine died from both feuding families, including Juan's grandmother and father.

After Frank and the medical team had stabilized the wounded, they searched the house, where they found Juan whimpering in his brother's arms. They were both in deep shock and terrified. Frank convinced Juan's relatives to permit him to take the boy to Catacamas. Frank bundled Juan up in a blanket, carried him to the vehicle, and with his team took the four-year-old boy down the mountain.

Juan was treated at the Good Samaritan Clinic. Frank and his team then transported Juan to the hospital in Juticalpa, where the doctors examined him, then referred him to a hospital in Tegucigalpa. The bullets had shattered Juan's leg. His injuries were so severe the only hope of saving his leg was to see a specialist in the capital city. At the hospital in Tegucigalpa, doctors operated to save Juan's leg. Even after surgery, there was no certainty he would walk again.

Predisan supervised Juan's recovery in the weeks that followed. When the cast was removed, he walked with a limp but soon regained strength and learned to walk normally, eventually running and jumping like little boys should. But his psyche suffered irreparable damage. At an age too young to be dealing with such issues, he wanted to know, "Why are there bad people in the world?"

Hearing a gunshot one day Juan told a caretaker, "That's how my grandmother and father died." Weeks later, Juan was reunited with his mother, who had separated from Juan's father and moved to the north coast.

Dr. Madrid had seen enough of the senseless violence in the mountain jungles. Not only were nine people killed in the recent attack, but the health of thousands of people in Olancho also came under attack. As a result of the battle, the two feuding families prepared for all out village war. Clinics in the region shut down again because of the feuds, funerals, and fear.

Meanwhile Dr. Madrid gathered a coalition of her own, to negotiate peace with the two families. She enlisted civic and religious leaders to come with her. Some leaders, however, were terrified to go into the mountain jungles where Dr. Madrid had been working for two and a half decades.

She contacted the mayor of Catacamas, asking him to talk with the gangs that aligned themselves with drug traffickers and cast a pall of fear over the once peaceful mountain region where the five Predisan clinics were located. The mayor either could not or would not go. Dr. Madrid went to the chief of police and asked, "Will you send a police force to face these armed men?"

The police chief decided he would not send a force or go himself. Dr. Madrid asked if the city would provide a car or police transport for them. No, she was told, all extra police cars were broken down, all extra drivers were "sick."

Some Predisan employees were also afraid of the escalating violence in the mountains. But Dr. Madrid had a small but fearless coalition of Predisan employees willing to go with her anywhere for the cause: to preach and to heal.

Dr. Madrid's fearless coalition included the following:

Don Gil, veteran Predisan driver, began each day in his driver's seat with an audible prayer for all those in the vehicle, with his forehead bowed and resting on the steering wheel. In the twenty years he'd driven through floodwaters and danger for Dr. Madrid, he had become family to her.

Frank Lopez had grown up in the Cuyamel River Valley where the clinics were being destroyed by drug running and feuding families. Frank knew most of the murder victims in the valley—some were childhood friends and cousins. He directed the work of five mountain clinics. Dr. Madrid called him her "cultural broker." He knew he had to calm Predisan employees, patients, and volunteers in the mountain clinics.

Juan Carrasco was the coordinator of spiritual development in the mountain area. Juan spent much of his time praying with people there, reading scripture, and encouraging.

Fernando Rodriguez was the president of the *Federation of Patronatos Locales*. Almost every village had a *patronato* or advocate. A close neighbor of one of the warring families, Fernando was a smart man in his mid-fifties with a good reputation who was trusted in the Cuyamel River Valley. The relaxed look of his brushed black wavy grey hair and shirt with four embroidered pockets belied his paranoia. When the killings began in 2009, he feared for his life, so on a few occasions he took refuge with friends in Catacamas.

Two other women went with the coalition: Dr. Madrid's brave young assistant and a local woman who said she was a friend of all the narcos.

The plan was to meet with the two groups separately at CEDECO, the clinic network headquarters in the mountains. Though the groups were identified with families and causes— one seemed bent on aligning with drug cartels and one seemed determined to defend their village from the cartels—both seemed rife with mixed motives. Many people were involved beyond those families, so the peacekeepers referred to the men of the Mendoza family and supporters as "Group A" and to the Salazar family and supporters as "Group B."

The Predisan peace coalition intended only to meet Group A, then return another day to meet with Group B. Both groups wanted to avenge the deaths of their family members. The Mendozas and Salazars planned a clash at the Cuyamel River between their villages to settle scores. If the coalition did not come quickly, the Cuyamel River would run with blood of the Mendozas and Salazars, more children would be left fatherless.

The peace coalition drove into the mountains, nearly reaching the site for the peace negotiation, but they were stopped by men with AK-47s, grenades, and two-way radios. An armed man entered the vehicle to accompany them to the next roadblock. They checked through three roadblocks and were told at the last one to wait at the Predisan mountain clinic headquarters, CEDECO.

They turned off the mountain road onto a path leading up a hill to the buildings of CEDECO. Hammocks hung from the rafters around the porch of the large brick building that served as a classroom and meeting space for clinic staff and church gatherings. The peace coalition got out of the car, used the rest rooms, then washed and cooled their faces after a hot drive through dusty, mountain roads. A thirty-foot tall tank supplied water to the facility. They waited at CEDECO headquarters for instructions from the armed men in Group A. They prayed over their strategy for averting a village war.

The coalition talked, prayed, and sat nervously waiting. Three hours after they had arrived, a man named Rodrigo rode up on a horse and greeted the group loudly.

"Finally you got here! Where have you been? We've been waiting for you! We are ready to attack them," Rodrigo said. He wore dark glasses and had an AK-47 strapped across his back.

Dr. Madrid thought but did not say, *Where have we been? We've been waiting here for three hours!*

Rodrigo instructed the group that they were to meet at the soccer field in the center of Las Delicias village. The group walked down the concrete steps behind the CEDECO buildings, descending through beds of colorful flowers shaded by palms and banana trees.

They exited the CEDECO property gate and walked a quarter mile to the meeting site, a tiny soccer field surrounded by trees, a few houses, and mountains in the distance. Makeshift, half-sized soccer goals matched the lumpy overgrown field. A lone donkey stood motionless in a corral nearby, dogs yapped, and mothers called their children inside; the normal sounds of their chatter and playing were absent. Most front doors of homes that normally remained opened throughout the village were closed and locked.

The coalition carried a cooler with cold drinks to give the men while they negotiated. They thought the chilled drinks would cool the emotions of the agitated men. If something did not change the course of this feud, a firefight would soon commence that could easily double the number of deaths in the region to one hundred.

As they walked along the dirt road from CEDECO to the soccer field, men with weapons from Group A loomed behind trees. The men treated the Predisan group as hostiles, as if their container of cool drinks contained an I.E.D.

When the peace coalition arrived at the soccer field, they watched as more armed men surrounded them. Dr. Madrid realized this was a dangerously impossible place to escape if gunfire erupted. Along the line of trees forming a shady perimeter around the field, the delegation put down their cooler. They sat on the rickety benches around the soccer field meant for use when watching "the beautiful game."

The delegation remained silent and tense as dozens of men pointed their guns at them. Most men wore camo to blend into the jungle undergrowth and ski masks to hide identities. Some were locals, others were mercenaries paid by the drug cartels.

Dr. Madrid did not have a handkerchief so she swiped her brow with her hand then wiped sweat on the side of her stylish jeans that she wore with a Predisan t-shirt and red high heels. She wondered how these guys wore ski masks in ninety-degree heat. The smell of sweaty fear hung in the air. Some of the lackeys who'd joined the fray were issued rifles but not trained to handle them; they lazily slumped the Kalashnikovs in the direction of the delegation. Did the armed men know whether the safety position on an AK-47 was up or down, and would they use the safety? Dr. Madrid's heart slammed in her chest the way yours would if a dozen men pointed Kalashnikovs at you at close range. The doctor had been trained in the Honduran military, but there was no page in the field manual titled, "How to stay calm while undisciplined thugs aim AK-47s at you."

In one way, however, the presence of the men comforted Dr. Madrid because she knew that they thought the place was secure and that they were in control. If they felt as if they were in control, maybe they wouldn't feel threatened and try to start something. Dr. Madrid noticed the armed men open their eyes wide when they saw the cold drinks in the coolers. Don Gil and Frank Lopez handed bottles of cold water and sodas to the armed men, who quickly uncapped and downed the drinks. The emotional temperature of the soccer grounds dropped a few degrees after they drank.

She didn't sign up for this when she moved to Catacamas. She steadied her trembling hands as she went over her written thoughts for the negotiation. The peacekeeping force came unarmed. So why had Group A come out to meet them with enough firepower to kill hundreds?

She wondered if she'd make it home alive. Her children and staff had worried about her going to the mountains to face feuding men, some with ties to drug cartels. Dr. Madrid and the Predisan staff knew what these violent men and their foes were capable of: forty-two murders in the Cuyamel River region of central Honduras. Over many years, the doctor had medically treated many of the men and their families. She had delivered and cared for children these men fathered. This day could turn into a terrible tragedy, so she didn't want to imagine what the inebriated, drug-fueled ones could easily do to her in a heartbeat.

Water and soda bottles lay in the grass all around them as the men finished their drinks. Village children would later fetch the bottles for re-use. Dr. Madrid's pulse quickened when she heard a vehicle approaching. Was it the other group coming to attack? She breathed deeply and tried to stay calm.

A green Toyota SUV roared up the road in front of them, drove onto the field, slammed on the brakes, and parked. Heavily armed men in camo, sunglasses, and ski masks exited the vehicle, then the leader, Julio, got out and walked across the grass toward the peace delegation. Two men in cowboy hats, jeans, button-down shirts, and designer cowboy boots walked on either side of Julio.

Standing in front of the delegation, Julio didn't ask them to talk, didn't greet them; he abruptly launched into an interrogation.

"¿lo que están haciendo ustedes aquí? What are you doing here?" Julio said, his voice booming. "This is our business! What do you hope to accomplish by coming here!"

The delegation sat quietly, wincing, but trying to remain calm during Julio's rant. They had practiced this, talked about how it would go. They did not count on so many men with AK-47s, the heat, complete vulnerability, the leader screaming and spitting threats at them. Julio carried for several minutes, sweat pouring down his shirt. He wore fatigues and had a pistol tucked in his pants.

Dr. Madrid knew who Julio was—a known killer, a mercenary. But he born and raised in the Cuyamel River Valley. He grew up with his cousin, Frank Lopez, of Predisan. As a teenager Julio had been happy and calm. Frank, Julio, and other teenagers in the

Cuyamel River Valley attended school together, played pick-up soccer matches with a tattered ball, celebrated fiestas, and did not drink alcohol—lots of coffee but no alcohol; they'd dance, talk, play, sing, eat tamales, and throw firecrackers at the pigs.

Then Julio got married as a teenager to a girl named Flora, who soon gave birth to a son. Julio abandoned Flora after he got her pregnant again. Flora gave birth to a second son and raised her children without their father.

In a neighboring village, a friend asked Julio to help him settle a score with another man. With machetes, Julio and his friend ambushed and killed the man and his cousin. Fearing a reprisal, Julio fled for Tegucigalpa, where he lived ten years; then after six years in the United States, he returned to Honduras.

Julio returned to Cuyamel and one day caught sight of his sons, now teenagers. He had no relationship with them, but soon after he returned, his first son was killed in a drunken machete fight with a group of boys. Julio began investigating who killed his son, then began a new reign of terror in the village by killing his son's best friend and hunting down any others who were present at the fight.

Later at a soccer match between village teams, a dispute arose between two families over a piece of land. Julio was friends with the Salazars, who controlled property another family wanted. Julio and his friends told the neighbors, the Mendoza family, to leave the land alone or someone would get killed. The leader of the Mendoza family said he had money in the deal and was not going to leave it alone. After the soccer game, Julio and the Salazars confronted the Mendozas and a gun battle erupted. Julio's younger son yelled, "If any Salazars die, I will kill every one of the Mendoza family members." As he was screaming those words, he was hit in the chest with a bullet; he fell to the ground and bled to death.

Julio had lost both his sons.

Though Julio was a friend to the Salazars, he believed they had shot the bullet that killed his second son. He amassed an army of fifteen men who attacked the Salazar family; half of Julio's men were killed in the battle. That was the battle when four-year-old Juan was shot in the leg.

Frank's cousin Julio asked the delegation again, *"¿qué estás haciendo aquí?* What are you doing here?!"

What was Frank Lopez doing here? He'd grown up here with Julio. But when Julio left, Frank followed his own dream to train as a community health care worker. Now Frank had come back to his own community that was falling apart. His wife was terrified he would not return, but Frank told her that he was not afraid to die. Frank's wife replied that Predisan would send her flowers but they could not bring him back from the dead.

And what was Dr. Madrid doing here? Frank Lopez and Julio were young boys when Dr. Madrid rode horseback up the mountains. She'd invested her life in these mountain villages.

What was the delegation doing here? Dr. Amanda talked first.

"My name is Dr. Amanda Madrid. I am the director of Predisan. We are a delegation that has come here to help facilitate reconciliation in the community. I know many of your families because I've been working here for twenty-five years. I know many of you have been hurt, relatives have died, and you have experienced a lot of pain. There has been a lot of bloodshed, but more killing will not bring your family members back. Instead, you can do something to honor them. I want you to know that God cares and we care."

"You care?" Julio asked.

"Yes, we care. God cares about you. That's why we're here."

"Oh, you people care? You only care because a university professor's son was killed!" Julio said. He was referring to the university rector named Dr. Julieta Castellanos, whose son was allegedly killed by police some believed were controlled by drug cartels.

"We do care. We don't know who's bad or good, but we do know violence and insecurity are preventing people from getting health care, and people are afraid to travel because you are threatening them on the roads."

"Where were you when my dad and my sons were killed?" Julio asked.

"We have been in these villages for many years, and we also knew your father and sons. We are very sorry they died. But killing more innocent people will not bring them back," Dr. Madrid said.

"You people in your churches pray, but you do nothing. You pray but that doesn't help. Your prayers inside your churches have not prevented this from happening!" Julio said.

A local pastor who had joined the coalition in Las Delicias apologized for the shortcomings of churches, but Julio did not acknowledge this apology. Julio gave Dr. Madrid a written list of the grievances against the other group. As they came closer and stood watching her read the grievances, Dr. Madrid smelled their sweating bodies in clothes not made for the heat. She sensed in the damp letter a deep odor of bitterness, fear, and grief as well as raw hatred.

Julio's grievances were about lives taken and disrespected by the Salazars. He blamed the death of his second son on the Salazars. The Salazars had irreligiously buried seven of Julio's men in a mass grave after a the gun battle that hurt four-year-old Juan.

Rodrigo, the husband of a health care worker, said "I'm not going to let them take over our village, steal our cows, and kill our sons," he said.

"Rodrigo," Dr. Madrid said, "you really need to stop acting like this. You are not a bad person. You are the husband of one of my nurses at Predisan, and you can't act like this! Your wife is a good woman. Think about your wife and your children! Put down your gun, Rodrigo. All of you, put down your guns."

Julio added, "The Salazars kill people for no reason, take property, and we're not going to let them do that."

"Predisan clinics are closed due to this violence and insecurity, schools are closed, people are dying—a woman in childbirth died when her family was afraid to take her to the hospital because of your roadblocks."

Rodrigo said, "We accept what you say, but the Salazars are loco, so we're going to be ready for them."

"I can't fix all the problems, but I want to help people heal physically and spiritually," Dr. Amanda said. "More bloodshed will never help, it will only make things worse. What will it take for you to have peace?"

"Will you talk to the other group—the Salazars?" Julio wanted to know.

"We're planning to meet with them another day," Dr. Amanda said.

"No, we can't wait till another day! We are ready to attack them today before they attack us," Julio said.

"Okay, okay—if we meet today with the other group, will you wait and not attack them?" Dr. Madrid said.

Julio and Rodrigo retreated from the coalition to talk for a long time. When they returned, they told Dr. Madrid that they agreed to wait, to let the delegation send men to Group B to find out if they would also be willing to talk. If Group B did talk, Group A agreed to send two delegates to Catacamas to sign a peace agreement. The delegation described a plan for Group A to sign the agreement at City Hall and Group B to sign at Good Samaritan Clinic, then a date for that signing day would be set so that peace could come again to the Cuyamel River Valley. Feeling the raging heat in the village, seeing the grenades hanging from the men's camo pants, the ski masks, the dozens of Kalashnikovs—she didn't know if these men could purge themselves of revenge and not shed blood.

After Group A and the peace delegation finished saying all they could in the heat on that soccer field, Don Gil sang a few hymns. Dr. Madrid gathered Julio and all of his men closer in a tighter circle. Men came from behind trees, still aiming their weapons. Julio instructed his men to lower their guns. Dr. Madrid put her hand on Julio's shoulder, and prayed for the men.

"Loving Father, these are your sons, and you love each one of them. You love each one of us. I believe you do not want us warring against one another but you want peace among brothers and sisters in every city and village. Holy God, bring your peace to this land and through the blood of Christ forgive us our trespasses. Help these two sides warring against each other to forgive. Help them again become a hopeful and loving community," Dr. Madrid prayed.

Julio calmed down during the prayer. Tears streamed from his eyes for the father and sons he had lost, for the grief that had turned to hatred that the doctor prayed would turn to forgiveness.

Dr. Madrid was not sure if Group B would meet. Group A was more connected to drug trafficking activities, but Group B was more hostile because the last death had been on their side, a brother of the family and one of the main leaders. Because of this hostility, the peacemakers were hesitant to drive the vehicle toward the houses of Group B higher up the mountain road in a village called Agua Caliente.

They decided to send two men—Don Gil and Fernando Rodriguez—up the road in the Predisan vehicle. When they got close to Agua Caliente, the men parked the truck and walked up the road cautiously, holding their hands above their heads as they approached the main house of the family of Group B. Their mission was to find out if they were willing to discuss a peace agreement as Group A had.

Meanwhile, the rest of the delegation walked back to CEDECO to rest and to prepare themselves for a second round of talks. They prayed and looked for Bible verses they could read at the second meeting. They had a two-way radio and were in communication with the two emissaries to Group B. They had another car in case the response was positive, and they would drive to meet the two advance men of the delegation.

Nearly an hour passed before Dr. Madrid received a call on her radio from Don Gil. The Salazars, Group B, wanted to meet in Agua Caliente. The delegation got in the small borrowed car, ascended the dirt road, and turned onto a smaller path with worn car tracks and grass in the middle. The property was so rich with vegetation, palms, banana plants, and rows of corn that they could not see a house.

They drove slowly down the path, past a few horses saddled and tied up to fence posts. Then Dr. Madrid saw the house where twenty men were gathered. Unlike Group A, they wore no ski masks and drove no fancy Toyota SUV. The driver parked the vehicle, and the rest of the coalition walked slowly to the front porch where the men were seated. Dr. Madrid noticed that some men dressed in *campesino* (farmer) daily wear—cowboy hats, boots, jeans—while others were wearing camo and holding weapons.

The angry, sweat-soaked men stood in bold relief to the beautiful land around them, resplendent with coconut palms, bougainvillea, lush grass, and a thriving fish pond down the hill from the house. The brick house had wood poles holding up the large front porch that provided shade for the meeting. The roof of the house was red tile, and smoke rose behind the house where women cooked for all the men rattling their machetes for war.

Young men brought chairs for the delegation members. As they were taking their seats, Dr. Madrid noticed one of the key leaders, Emilio, had at least three weapons strapped across his body and grenades clipped to his belt. A family member in Tegucigalpa provided arms for Group B. Emilio's brother had been killed, and he blamed Rodrigo of Group A for killing him. The intention of the Salazars, Group B, was to avenge the death of Emilio's brother. They had no plans to meet the Mendozas, Group A, except in battle.

Emilio was aggressive and vile, as Julio of Group A had been. He drunkenly waved a gun, saying he would avenge the blood of his brother. Another of Emilio's brothers, Diego, quietly listened with a determined look of agreement. Group B showed more aggression toward the delegation, standing up and pointing in the faces of Dr. Madrid and the other members. They did not listen when the delegation tried to talk. They refused to put down their weapons, instead threatening the delegation, including Dr. Madrid, at gunpoint.

Dr. Madrid swallowed hard, but she had been around guns many times in the military in Tegucigalpa, had been caught in the middle of a firefight along the Patuca River, had run down armed thieves who stole a Predisan vehicle, and earlier that day had looked down the barrels of many other guns. But with a gun pointed in her face she still felt a powerful impulse to flee.

She pondered how to convince Emilio to put down his gun and talk. The doctor asked if she could talk by phone to Emilio's supporter and main leader, Maynor, who was in Tegucigalpa at the time. Perhaps Maynor would be more reasonable; perhaps he could talk to Emilio and convince his men to put down their weapons. One of the Salazars called Maynor on his cell phone and after a few minutes gave the phone to Dr. Madrid, who explained the goal of the coalition, then she listened as Maynor explained the Salazar grievances.

Three hours passed. They negotiated, relayed grievances by phone, and prayed. The coalition had now accomplished one of its goals in working toward peace: they had heard grievances directly from the Mendozas and Salazars.

After the coalition had recorded all grievances of Group B, Dr. Madrid asked Group B a final question.

"Will you sign a peace agreement?"

Group B discussed among themselves what they would do. They did not agree that they would sign a peace agreement. They would have to consult further with Maynor.

Meanwhile, Emilio's avenging tone escalated rather than subsided.

"I will kill whoever killed my brother, and I will have no compassion," Emilio said. He even spat out the numbers of men—women and children as well—that his men were going to slaughter.

"Don't be crazy!" Dr. Amanda said to Emilio, "because the devil is who got you like this. You are not a bad person. You are a good person. Killing will not help you or make you feel better. It will only make things worse."

Dr. Madrid had known Emilio and Diego since they were young boys. She had treated them in the rural clinics.

"I knew your father," Dr. Madrid told the young men, "I knew your uncle, I've known all of you to be good people. I've treated some of you in the clinics. I remember when you were kids, and now you're telling me you're going to kill all these people? You have been in some of our youth activities and now you tell me you are merciless killers?"

Dr. Madrid had a cauldron of her own boiling, an anger at the constant stream of men—and sometimes women—who had allowed others with their craziness to determine their actions.

The doctor stood up and moved closer to Emilio, leaning toward him with her finger jabbing the air in front of his chest. She was yelling now. *"Baja tu rifle!* Lay down your rifle!"

She narrowed her focus on Emilio. *"Mírame!* Look at me! *Escucha!* Listen!" Dr. Madrid said. She became aware of her screaming and shifted to a motherly tone.

"You have heard God's word so many times, Emilio. You are not a killer."

Emilio said nothing. His eyebrows wrinkled.

Dr. Madrid continued. *"Usted es un buen hombre.* You are a good person." At the words, *"un buen hombre,"* a look of perplexed disbelief displaced Emilio's angry expression.

Emilio lowered his gun and put it down against a chair on the porch.

Dr. Madrid hugged Emilio, and he cried on her shoulder.

Emilio pulled back from Dr. Madrid and looked at her eye to eye. Tears streamed down his face.

"Thank you for telling me that I am good," Emilio said. "I have not heard that in a long time."

They all sat down on the porch and prayed. The coalition, led by Don Gil, sang Christian hymns, then they read from the Bible the texts that would cause them to remember to love and not hate, even their enemies. They read texts like Matthew 5:43-44 where Jesus said: "You've heard it said, love your neighbor and hate your enemy, but I tell you, love your enemy and pray for those who persecute you."

Some had never heard that Bible reading before. Love your neighbor, yes, but love and pray for your enemy? How could Emilio and Diego pray for enemies who killed their brother?

After they prayed, sang songs, and read the Bible, Dr. Madrid told the men a story about the time when she was in another village and a violent dispute arose among the men. This dispute is the same, she told them.

"You are fighting to find out who has the biggest balls! Why didn't you tell me before all the killing? I could have settled this war with a knife and a scale!" Dr. Madrid said.

The men tried to remain serious but their gruff scowls broke, and they laughed. One of the men said between laughs, "I was there that day! I remember you said that!"

"Then why didn't you realize this is what's happening here, too?" Dr. Madrid said.

At the end Dr. Madrid embraced each of the Salazars and their friends. Reminding them of the date for the peace agreement signing, she said goodbye, and the coalition left Agua Caliente, driving back through Las Delicias and back to Catacamas.

Both groups had given Dr. Madrid a list of grievances. The peace coalition quickly returned and over the next few days typed up letters from their memory of the events and the written lists of grievances of Group A and B. Both groups gave their word they would come to sign the documents.

Dr. Madrid had mixed feelings about the signing. On the one hand, the doctor believed the impossible could happen: a peace agreement would be enacted and the constant threat of reprisals and insecurity would be transformed into a more lasting peace as the groups began to work on making amends toward each other's grievances. On the other hand, Dr. Madrid had seen, at close range, their firepower and seething anger, so she did not want violence to spill over into Catacamas. Discussing grievances and bringing the feuding men to Catacamas had certain risks: what if they saw relatives or friends of their enemies in town? Was the delegation bringing danger to Predisan by signing the agreement at their hospital site? Would it endanger others at Predisan?

Because of the unexpected and violent things the groups could do, the peace delegation arranged two different sites so the groups could sign the document separately. The biggest question of all, as they waited for the two separate days of signing, was whether or not the two groups would even show up.

Miraculously, both groups attended their individual signing ceremonies. The mayor of Catacamas agreed to attend the signings and hosted one meeting at city hall. Dr. Madrid and the delegation attended both meetings. Predisan hosted the other group at the Good Samaritan Clinic. Each group did not know when or where the other group signing ceremony would take place.

Both Group A and B agreed to basic principles of peace in a letter typed for them in Spanish then signed by Dr. Madrid and more than a dozen participants in the peace process, including municipal, religious, and community leaders. The agreements both groups signed were nearly identical. The grievances against each other were worded into agreements and amends that could bring peace to the Cuyamel River Valley.

Group B wanted money for the damages to three homes on the Salazar ranch. They had brought with them to the signing an attorney and a journalist.

Group A wanted money for proper burial of Julio's men who died in an ambush.

Both listed property such as cars they expected the other group to compensate them for damaging.

Both groups agreed to seek peace with great sincerity.

Both groups would not provide support for any person trying to destroy the peace.

Groups A and B agreed not to attack the other.

They both agreed to stay off each other's land.

Both would not stop vehicles along the road as a security measure, which only frightened people, adding a general feeling of insecurity in the village.

They agreed to loosen their ties to the mercenaries who joined each of the groups and provided guns for their battles.

They agreed in principle to the wisdom of establishing a military police post in the Cuyamel River Valley to keep the peace.

They signed an agreement to disarm, except for legally permitted guns. Finally, the Salazars and Mendozas had agreed to lay down their guns. Still, Dr. Madrid wondered how long the peace would last.

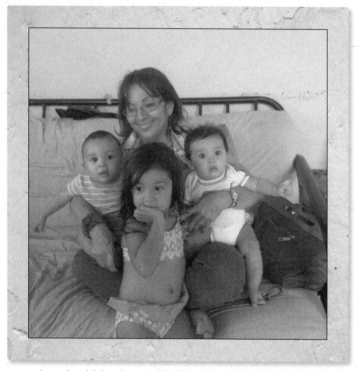

*Amanda with her three grandchildren (from left) Anthony David Madrid Mendez, Leyla Rebekah Folger, and Jonathan Lucas Folger.*

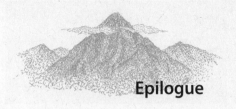

# CAN PEACE LAST?

**Dr. Amanda Madrid and the peace coalition prevented more bloodshed between the Salazars and Mendoza families and their recruits. Into this hot cauldron of hatred,** Dr. Madrid and the coalition entered, muttering prayers that God would somehow miraculously cause these men to lay down their guns. Perhaps someday the *fútbol* pitch might be used again for its intended purpose, villagers would gather for *fiestas* and *quinceañeras*, and the network of clinics could thrive again.

The peace coalition had succeeded, for the time being. The peace agreement lasted from October 2011 until April 2012, when the Salazars, Group B, killed a relative of Julio from Group A. The Mendozas retaliated with reprisal killings and stole a vehicle of Group B.

Then on August 15, 2012 Julio and a mercenary army of drug lords stormed the Salazars' ranch. The once peaceful ranch with healthy crops, a fish pond, and children playing—where Dr. Madrid met with Group B—was now surrounded by mercenaries of Group A on yet another reprisal mission. This was the place where Dr. Madrid told Emilio that God loves him, that he was a good person.

Fernando Rodriguez, the middle-aged man from Agua Caliente who helped Dr. Madrid and the coalition broker the peace deal, called Dr. Madrid from a perch high in a tree during the attack.

"Ten vehicles full of men came and blew up the Salazar house. They are looking for anyone sympathetic with saving the village from the drug lords. This may be the last time I talk to you," Fernando said. The Mendoza group blew a hole in the roof with a grenade, shattering roofing tiles across the yard, and they burned other houses of Salazar family members who lived close by.

"I'm going to get you help, Fernando. Be very careful and stay out of the open. Where is your family?"

"They are hiding with me in the jungle," Fernando said.

Diego also escaped to "run like a fox and burrow in like an armadillo," and await his chance to avenge the blood of his brother. The attackers had killed Diego's brother, leaving his body amid the shattered roofing tiles and burning buildings. Seeking information about others who had escaped, the attackers beat an elderly neighbor. Horses had been shot and killed, some still tied to fence posts and slumped over.

Fernando chose not to join sides and seek revenge, but he returned to peace efforts, staying in contact with Dr. Madrid, attempting with her to work with authorities to bring criminals to justice in the Cuyamel River Valley.

Shortly after hearing about the attack on the Salazar ranch and the killings, Dr. Madrid was at a government function, attended by the United States Ambassador to Honduras. A North American hospital administrator working with Dr. Madrid on community health and conflict transformation attended the function with Dr. Madrid.

"I am not an American—I'm a Mayan from Honduras—but I host four hundred United States citizens annually in the organization I direct. My children are married to North Americans," Dr. Madrid told the official. "We need your help in the mountains in Central Honduras." The doctor made it clear to the ambassador how the drug trade has destabilized the region and devastated community health.

After their brief meeting, the ambassador worked with her staff and Honduran officials to call the head of police in Tegucigalpa, *El Tigre,* who had been Dr. Madrid's superior officer in the military years before. *El Tigre* ordered a brigade of police from Catacamas to the mountains to secure the area around Agua Caliente.

With the backing of police, several of the peace coalition and Predisan directors went along to secure CEDECO and reassure the mountain clinic staff. They were more afraid than ever before, because paid mercenaries had come in force and remained in the Cuyamel River Valley with heavy firepower. They could easily ambush Predisan and police vehicles as they entered the villages.

When the police hesitated to continue into the mountains, stopping miles short of where the violent men had been spotted, Dr. Madrid said, "You're job is not to go and pick up dead bodies. Your job is to protect citizens!" Dr. Madrid said.

When the attacking force from Group A got word that the police were coming, they scattered to hiding places in the surrounding villages. Scratchy reports from police positioned around the region blared from the police commander's two-way radio. The police did not know the region well and relied on Dr. Madrid and other Predisan directors to relay information about how they might find the mercenaries and take them in for questioning.

When police reached one of the mountain medical clinics, the police commander told Amanda he needed her help to locate the armed men. As they walked together, the commander had his two-way radio in his hand. Trying to re-attach the radio to his belt, the commander stumbled, and his hand swiped across the AK-47 strapped to his back. The gun fired.

He looked around with surprise. He knew it was his, could feel it pop on his back. He looked down and saw a hole in his boot. He took off his boot and it was full of blood. The commander cried out, "I shot myself!"

Dr. Madrid jumped into the police vehicle with the commander, and the driver sped toward the hospital down the mountain. As they drove Dr. Madrid said, "Take off your sock and let me see your foot."

Dr. Madrid looked at the wound and it was superficial.

"Turn the car around," she told the driver.

The driver kept going, to reach the first clinic or hospital they could find.

"What should I do, Colonel?" the driver asked.

"This thing hurts!" the commander said.

"Turn the car around!" Dr. Madrid screamed. "He's not hurt badly."

"What?" the commander asked.

"The bullet did not hit the bone. You are fine. It just grazed you and tore soft flesh."

The driver turned around and they drove back to the clinic. The driver and a few policemen standing around the clinic property carried the commander inside, where the doctor administered an anti-tetanus shot, antibiotics, pain medicine, and wrapped his foot with gauze.

"How long until I can walk again, doctor?" the commander asked.

"A few minutes. Put your boot on and walk," Dr. Madrid said.

The commander led a security meeting for the villages at CEDECO in the large meeting room, and the police established outposts around the Cuyamel River Valley to secure the area.

Even though the police went to the Cuyamel River Valley, they did not find the armed men, because everyone was hiding or on the run. Another cycle of panic returned to the region. Clinics and schools closed. People feared for their lives. Even with police presence, mountain residents wondered if they were imposters.

Police gathered evidence, testimonies, submitted it to prosecutors and eventually Julio from Group A and Emilio from Group B were captured. Both these key leaders were tried in Honduran courts for their crimes, convicted, and sent to prison. Police also captured and put on trial one of the mercenaries for the drug lords, and he was convicted and sent to prison.

With those three violent men in prison, the people in the mountains feel safer. In early 2013, $2 million in arms, drugs, and cash was confiscated in the mountains surrounding the Cuyamel River Valley. *El Tigre* headed the military police force that seized the cache of drugs, money, and weapons. Dr. Madrid had not seen him in years. She asked if he remembered the day they met. *El Tigre* laughed. Of course he remembered the female medical officer who was not afraid to confront a lieutenant.

I went with Dr. Amanda Madrid to the mountain region and CEDECO when she spoke to a large gathering of health care workers from the five mountain clinics. I watched her calm their fears. They prayed, strategized, read scripture, sang songs, laughed, and grieved losses one more time together.

"We live in an imperfect world and bad things happen to us, but Predisan has come to preach and heal," Dr. Madrid said. "We will continue to do that. God does not take us away from this world—not yet. We do not escape the realities of the world around us but seek to change the reality in the name of Christ. Fixing the broken world is the work of God. Our work is to make ourselves available to God and others to serve. Serving God doesn't mean we won't get injured or sick, suffer or die. When we serve Christ, we will suffer like Christ. My life is forever sheltered in God, no matter what happens to me. I'm not afraid to die."

After Dr. Madrid's visit, the health care workers re-opened the five mountain clinics and went back to work saving lives in the Cuyamel River Valley.

# Reading in Action

1. See www.gregrtaylor.com for more photos, stories, reviews, and ideas about what you've read.

2. Buy your books at a local bookstore. You may have to order it through the store the first time, but this helps booksellers see the book among thousands of inventory choices they have, and purchase more for customers.

3. Tell your friends about the book and encourage them to buy it at bookstores as well. Giving the book away is kind of you, but it also prevents your friends from contributing as you did to Predisan. It also prevents you from telling others about it when you want to re-read a passage or use it in a book club. For every book sold, about $3 goes to Predisan and Dr. Madrid.

4. Send a Honduran Child to School for One Year. Buy 100 books for your church or organization and the proceeds will be enough to send a child to school for an entire year. Contact Leafwood Publishers.

5. Suggest *Lay Down Your Guns* to a friend, bookstore, public radio station for a phone interview, book club (see questions on later page), library, missionaries, high school or college class, church, your doctor or those in the medical field.

6. Write a review for your blog, local newspaper, Facebook, Amazon, or send to a magazine or other web site. Feel free to critique the book strongly as well. The author is not looking for accolades but for the ups and downs of the book to be discussed and readers to be inspired.

7.  Check to see if *Lay Down Your Guns* is in your local library. If not, please donate a copy to your local library or suggest to the library that they add *Lay Down Your Guns*. Ask your friends and family in other states to also do this.

8.  Host a book signing at a local bookstore, your church, school or organization and invite Dr. Madrid and/or Greg Taylor to come and speak and sign books.

9.  Make a tax-deductible donation to Predisan

www.predisan.org
www.youtube.com/predisan
www.facebook.com/predisan
www.twitter.com/predisan

US phone 770-955-1512

Mailing address:
PREDISAN-USA, INC.
Post Office Box 72618
Marietta, GA  30007
EMAIL: info@predisan.org

10.  Go to Honduras. Medical and Surgical Brigades are a vital part of Predisan's outreach to the people of Honduras. Medical professionals of all kinds are needed. Please contact us to explore ways to connect your expertise or your group's expertise with the great needs in Honduras.

# PREDISAN means
## "to preach and to heal"

The name "Predisan" comes from two Spanish words: "predicar" (to proclaim) and "sanar" (to heal). These words are used in Luke 9:2, when Jesus sends his disciples out "... to proclaim the kingdom of God and to heal the sick." Predisan exists "to proclaim and to heal."

Predisan concentrates on three services: Healthcare, Spiritual Outreach/Formation, and Community Development. Since 1986 Predisan has been training and empowering Hondurans to share the love of Jesus, provide health care, addiction treatment, and community health.

Predisan employs about eighty Hondurans who equip and empower thousands of local leaders in Community Health Committees that collaborate with Predisan to sustain physical, spiritual, social, economic and environmental wellness.

Predisan focuses on the most marginal and unprotected Hondurans, especially those who are, in geographic and economic terms, at the greatest risk.

The centers for services include the following: Predisan Family Health Center and Good Samaritan Clinic in central Catacamas, one clinic in the rural suburbs of Catacamas, five clinics in remote mountain villages, and the CEREPA addiction treatment center in Catacamas.

Predisan serves more than 53 remote mountain villages from mobile mountain clinics.

Predisan is a non profit 501(c)(3) corporation registered in the U. S. as Predisan USA, Inc. and a non-profit corporation registered in Honduras as Asociacion Hondurena Predicar y Sanar (MISSION PREDISAN)

# Book Club Questions

1.  What feelings and thoughts did you have when you first learned Dr. Amanda Madrid was not only a doctor but also fighting a battle against drug cartels?

2.  How is the approach Dr. Madrid is taking different from the role of governments in preventing drug trafficking and use? Does one or the other seem to be working? Would you have the courage to face what might be parallel situations where you live?

3.  What connections do you see between Dr. Madrid's childhood stories and the path she chose to medical school, military training, and founding an addiction treatment center?

4.  How does Amanda deal with conflict throughout her life? In what ways does she too have to learn to lay down her guns? In particular, what happens in the story of her church "canceling her rights" and her family inheritance story that show how she laid down her guns?

5. What experiences prepared Dr. Madrid for facing armed men, or is there anything that can prepare someone for such a confrontation?

6. What did you enjoy or not enjoy about the book? How is the book unique from any other book you've read? How would you describe the story if someone in an airport or coffee shop saw you reading it and asked about it?

7. How did prayer influence Dr. Madrid's decisions early in her life and later?

# Acknowledgements

Dr. Madrid wishes to thank her mother, Maria Antonia, Eric and Linda King, all of the Predisan staff and board members in North and Central America, her children, Bartola, Fide, and Marcos, and grandchildren, Leyla, David, Jonathan.

Greg Taylor wishes to thank the following people who helped make the book a reality:

Dr. Amanda Madrid—You told me more than you ever expected, dredged up memories your subconscious mind only knew and perhaps you'd prefer to forget, but you told your story with honesty and love for every person who crosses your path, from your loving mother Maria Antonia to the most heinous of criminals you helped remove from the mountain jungles. Thank you for the dozens of personal conversations, and the hundreds of conversations by Skype, phone, and email. Your patience had no end, and one of my favorite emails from you was when your Spanish-English spell checker changed "spinal cord injury" to "Spinach Córdoba injure," which sounds tasty. Your story of courage, healing, and love for your fellow Hondurans captivated me, and I believe it will captivate readers and change the way they see God, the world, and themselves.

Linda King—*Lay Down Your Guns* would not exist without your vision, financial support from you and your husband, Eric, and the persistent drive to make the book worthy of the story and the legacy of Dr. Amanda Madrid.

Leonard Allen—Your confidence in me as a writer and cohort in publishing upholds me when I'm in the midst of redlined drafts and feel like quitting. Over a decade of work together, you have been my publisher, friend, and mentor.

Jill Taylor—You encouraged me to launch my writing career in 2000 when, led by your faith in God, you told me in the kitchen in Uganda to go and report on a mass murder in Kanungu, eight hours drive into the unknown. With each story I tell, you insist that it be precise and "a good story well told." Your sense for flow, sequence, and readability make my stories come alive in ways I could never accomplish alone. You are my best friend, and you tell me the truth.

Anna Taylor—My daughter, you are a courageous and adventurous young woman. Thank you for traveling with me to Honduras and helping me conduct interviews, take photos, write captions, and finish that jar of Nutella. Your grasp of Spanish increased what we could absorb in our research for this book and made it much better. Like Amanda, you are a middle child with strong character, and it serves you well in life. You, Ashley, and Jacob all inspire me with your lives and your love. I love you, mi Anita.

Wendy Call—As an early structural editor, you took a half-baked manuscript I thought was decent and showed me I had a lot of restructuring yet to accomplish and many more drafts to write. You turned up the heat on the structural changes that make it not only readable but a story anyone can wrap their minds around, even as they are amazed by its enormity and truth.

Isaac Alexander—Your original art for the cover was "just what the doctor ordered." Thank you for coming through on a short deadline for a big assignment. I've appreciated your artistic talents for twenty-five years.

Predisan-Honduras staff—You allowed me to interview for background stories of Predisan. You are part of an amazing organization that from top to bottom does "preach and heal": Marcio Matamoros, Keydy Flores, Martha Ponce, Hector Tejeda, Emelina Zúniga, Frank Lopez (you told the truth), Hector Gil

Martinez (thank you for driving us, your courage, and for your prayer on the steering wheel), Carlos Bonilla (you, Teresa, and my daughter Anna translated when I couldn't understand), Irene Ramirez, Marta Núñez, Eda Martinez, Martha Rivera, Jorge Alberto Gonzales Garcia, Elda Atanacia Hernández, Orlando Guifarro, Teresa Mejia, Juan Carrasco, Karla Abertina Posantes, Dunia Mendez Núñez, Gilberto Guifarro Montescleoca (thank you for hosting us on your beautiful land).

Predisan board members, United States staff, and supporters including Justin Myrick, Doris Clark, Joey Potter, Hugo Fruehauf, Paul and Katherine Evanson, Sharon Kemp, Kyle Huhtanan, Linda Trevathan, Linda Clark, Shane Jackson, Jeff and Dana Nicholson, Dr. Gary Harne, and Karen Rhodes—Thank you for granting interviews, reading early drafts, providing details about Predisan, and insisting on precision in the story. You provide the means and support that have made Predisan a growing international model for community health care that continues to follow the heart of Jesus' great commission and great commands: to love and heal and make disciples.

Dr. Madrid's family including Roger Madrid, Rebekah Folger Madrid, Marcos Madrid, Bartola Madrid, Fide Madrid Jones— You allowed me to look into your personal lives and trusted me there, and I appreciate your spirit of truth and humility. Barty, you were a gracious hostess and tireless and dependable source of information during a year of seemingly endless fact-checking.

Jim Shepard—Your ink drawings of the mountains, of a two-spire cathedral like the one in La Jigua, inspire but do not overpower the reader's imagination.

Zach Mason—Your piece on Toms vs. latrines was very helpful.

Blair A. Goforth—Thank you for the photo of Dr. Madrid's family.

Debbie Taylor—Your love of reading good stories inspired me to write stories you, Jill, and others want to read. You have a great eye for good photography. Thank you for your work on images and the book's readability.

Leafwood Publishers—Working at what I believe to be the best medium-size publishing company in the world, the following competent, creative, and professional staff and contractors are an author's dream team: Duane and Tammy Anderson, Ryan Self, Phil Dosa, Lettie Morrow, Seth Shaver, and Gary Myers.

Linda Clark, Robert D. Garland, Mark Manassee, Gilberto Guifarro Montescleoca, Hugo Fruehauf, Linda Trevathan, Cliff Fullerton, Mike Miller, Charlotte Taylor (I felt your prayers, Mom. I also know you read some of the book aloud to Dad, so thanks to Terrel Taylor, too), Toby Taylor, Linda King, Brooks Davis, Jill Taylor—Thank you for reading early manuscripts, encouraging me to press on, and powerful endorsements of Dr. Amanda Madrid. Anyone who reads early drafts is a saint. I hope you still have energy to read the final book.

Terri Taylor, Brent Taylor (thanks for 1964), Debbie French, Toby Taylor—Thank you for your love, sense of humor, and attempts to keep your youngest brother humble.

Aunt Becky Davis—I read you a few pages of an early draft while you were dying in a hospital bed in Oklahoma. Aunt Becky, your attention to my words and your laugh or chagrin at certain points in the reading inspired me to continue on, even when re-writing was excruciating and exhausting.

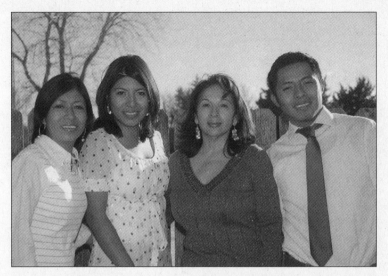

*Dr. Madrid with her children (from left) Bartola, Fide, Marcos. Madrid family*

Dr. Amanda Madrid is the Honduran founding medical director of Mission Predisan in Catacamas, Honduras.

She holds an M.D. degree from the National University of Honduras, a master's in International Public Health and a doctorate in International Public Health from Loma Linda University in California, and has had advanced training in addiction treatment.

She has served for 25 years with Mission Predisan, a Christian mission providing physical healing and spiritual hope at eight clinic facilities in Eastern Honduras. She is the founder of CEREPA, a Predisan ministry, which is the only comprehensive, Christian, in-patient addiction treatment center in Honduras.

She has received numerous honors including the Christian Service Award at the Pepperdine Bible Lectures, as 2008 Alumnus of the Year by the Loma Linda University School of Public Health, and in 2009 with a Crystal Globe award for service in world missions by Missions Resource Network.

Dr. Madrid served for three years as an adjunct faculty member at Oklahoma Christian University while working with Predisan-USA in fund-raising and development.

She was professor for Universidad Peruana Union in Peru, teaching addictive behaviors and program development.

She recently returned to live in Honduras and serve once again as Predisan's executive director, overseeing the medical work of the Good Samaritan Clinic, CEREPA and Predisan's seven mountain and barrio clinics.

Dr. Madrid has worked in fifteen countries on four continents, and is fluent in Spanish and English. She is a frequent consultant regarding medical care and public health. Most recently, she served as a medical program evaluator in Madagascar and Indonesia.

Dr. Madrid has three children, all graduates of Oklahoma Christian University, and three grandchildren.

# About the Author

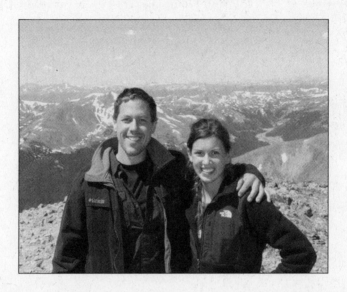

Greg R. Taylor with his daughter, Anna, who traveled to Honduras with him to assist with Spanish and research for the book.

Greg lives with his wife, Jill, and their three children, Ashley, Anna, and Jacob, in Broken Arrow, Oklahoma. Greg writes true stories that inspire readers to live justly, humbly, and mercifully. Contact the author at www.gregrtaylor.com